Stories in Midwifery:
Reflection, Inquiry, Action

Stories in Midwifery: Reflection, Inquiry, Action
Third Edition

Allison Cummins, Katharine Gillett, Karen McLaughlin,
Loretta Musgrave and Jessica Wood

ELSEVIER

Elsevier Australia. ACN 001 002 357
(a division of Reed International Books Australia Pty Ltd)
Tower 1, 475 Victoria Avenue, Chatswood, NSW 2067

ISBN: 978-0-7295-4455-9

Notice

Practitioners and researchers must always rely on their own experience and knowledge in evaluating and using any information, methods, compounds or experiments described herein. Because of rapid advances in the medical sciences, in particular, independent verification of diagnoses and drug dosages should be made. To the fullest extent of the law, no responsibility is assumed by Elsevier, authors, editors or contributors for any injury and/or damage to persons or property as a matter of products liability, negligence or otherwise, or from any use or operation of any methods, products, instructions, or ideas contained in the material herein.

National Library of Australia Cataloguing-in-Publication Data

A catalogue record for this book is available from the National Library of Australia

Content Strategists: Libby Houston and Dorothy Chiu
Content Project Manager: Shubham Dixit
Edited by Jo Crichton
Proofread by Tim Learner
Cover by Gopalakrishnan Venkatraman
Typeset by Aptara
Printed in China by 1010

Last digit is the print number: 9 8 7 6 5 4 3 2 1

Contents

Contents

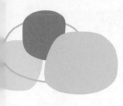

About the authors

Allison Cummins is a midwifery academic who is passionate about education and research. Allison is the Head of Midwifery at the University of Newcastle where she is implementing a new innovative curriculum. Allison makes an outstanding contribution to student learning through innovative subject design, embedding transitional workshops, whole-of-program coordination and co-design of curriculum. Allison has built a body of research around midwifery models of care and graduate transitions. Her renowned reputation for research in this specific area has led to national and international research opportunities. Through internal and external service and engagement, Allison has become a recognised leader in midwifery. She is a Midwifery Director on the Board for the Australian College of Midwives, current Chair of the Trans-Tasman Midwifery Education Consortium, and a member of the Quality Maternal Newborn Care Research Alliance. Allison is an Associate Editor of the midwifery journal *Women and Birth International (WOMBI)* that publishes relevant research on all matters that affect women and birth.

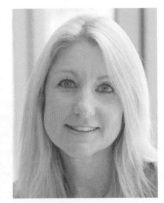

Katharine Gillett is a practising midwife on the Mid-North Coast and midwifery lecturer at the University of Newcastle. Katharine has a PhD in Creative Writing and is interested in how midwives and midwifery students can use poetry as part of a deeper reflective process, to help understand the universality of personal experience, and bring focus to the emotional work of midwifery.

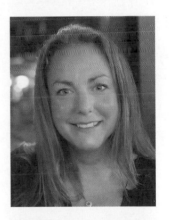

Karen McLaughlin is a midwifery academic and researcher who is passionate about midwifery and educating the next generation of midwives. Karen is a lecturer in Midwifery at the University of Newcastle and a Clinical Midwife Specialist practising in the Hunter New England Local Health District. Karen is contributing to student learning through the use of innovative teaching techniques and communication training. Karen's body of research includes antenatal asthma management and the role of midwives in antenatal asthma management and is now recognised nationally and internationally as an expert in this field. Karen has a passion for qualitative research methodologies and continues to build her body of research using these.

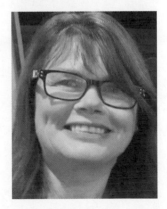

Loretta Musgrave is the Course Director of the Graduate Diploma of midwifery at the University of Technology, Sydney. With dual registration as both a registered midwife and a nurse, Loretta has over 27 years of clinical experience in the public healthcare system. Loretta has extensive experience in all areas of midwifery and has held leadership and management roles. Loretta completed her PhD in 2023 with the Faculty of Medicine at the University of Sydney. Her research interest includes life-course approaches to reproductive health and using mHealth as a behaviour change intervention for women of reproductive age.

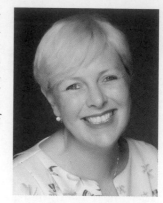

Jessica Wood is a midwifery lecturer and early career researcher at the University of Newcastle. With a background in both nursing and midwifery, Jessica has a strong interest in how innovative learning methods can be used to enhance learning experiences in tertiary education to improve the student experience. Jessica completed her PhD in 2021 which focused on the implementation of virtual reality simulation as a teaching method for midwifery students when learning neonatal resuscitation. Jessica is interested in exploring how new technologies and teaching methods can be used to enhance clinical skills learning and education among nurses, midwives, students and consumers.

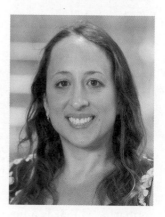

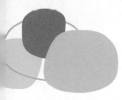# Acknowledgements

Acknowledgements and gratitude go to all the participants who contributed their time and freely told their stories. These contributions will enhance the development, knowledge and professionalism of midwives and other maternity health professionals when caring for women and families. The editors would also like to acknowledge Christine Catling and Rosemarie Hogan who contributed to the first and second editions of *Stories in Midwifery*.

Ashleigh Anning
Emma Bosker
Katie Burnett
Elise Campbell
Trish Crampton
Nikki Collins
Malika Elizabeth
Kaitlin Ellis
Tamara Ellis
Scott Ellis
Sandra Emerson
Robyn Evans
Cassandre Hall
Amy Hannaford
Ali Homer
David Homer
Sarah Jeffers

Jordan Lehmann
Leona McGrath
Jane McMurtrie
Vanessa Murphy
Emma Martine Ndenzako
Karolina Petrovska
Anke Reitter
Melanie Shilbury
Leia Sidery
Sheryl Sidery
Ella Smeets
Simon Smith
Kathryn Solanki
Sabera Turkmani
Christine Turner
Kate Williams
Namira Williams

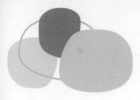# About this resource

Overview

This resource presents an in-depth look at the midwifery profession and the services provided by midwives. The stories are told from the perspectives of mothers, fathers and midwives, and are real-life experiences. From these personal experiences, readers will have the opportunity to reflect on the story and gain insight into topics.

The aim of this book is to provide the reader with a unique way of learning. In place of a standard text-book, this book encourages exploration of a topic beyond the confines of its pages. It is quite similar to the way we learn in everyday life: we listen, reflect on the information, investigate the topic further and ultimately develop an understanding and greater appreciation of a subject.

Using the resource

This book is designed for people who are interested in all aspects of midwifery. This can range from those undertaking certificate-level qualifications to under-graduate degrees and post-graduate studies. This resource is useful and informative for students from disciplines such as midwifery, nursing and medicine, or those undertaking any course that involves caring for women and their babies.

The book can be used in more than one way: as a teaching tool to facilitate students in researching a topic, or within a tertiary education setting where students have a more self-directed exploratory approach.

It is expected that this resource will be used online so that the reader may watch and listen to the stories of the participants. Alternatively, the transcripts of the stories can be read within the hard copy version of the book.

Structure of the resource

Using stories to relay information is a powerful way of learning. Relating information to actual events and experiences of people allows for a higher likelihood of knowledge retention. It personalises and humanises the story, so that the reader can link the topic to a person, instead of recalling words on a page. This way of learning engages the listener, allows for reflection and promotes an authentic learning experience.

Each chapter focuses on a particular aspect of midwifery/mother experience. Among others, these range from the experience of a homebirth to that of an emergency caesarean section. Clinicians (midwives and obstetricians) also provide input into other topics such as perinatal mental health, assisted reproductive techniques and caring for women having a vaginal breech birth. Within each chapter are a number of headings that guide the reader to explore the topic.

REFLECTION

The reader is asked to think widely about what they have listened to and/or read. The questions in this section will guide and stimulate reflective thinking.

INQUIRY

This section widens the topic for the reader by providing questions and further resources to guide learning.

ACTION

The reader is asked to apply their knowledge of a topic within the boundaries of their own midwifery practice.

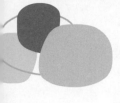

Inclusive language statement

The authors recognise and acknowledge that individuals have diverse gender identities. In this book the terms woman, mother and father have been used in accordance with the voices of the participants featured. The use of these terms is not meant to exclude those who give birth and do not identify as women. Language is changing to ensure inclusion and at times the authors have used the word parent to avoid gendering birth and those who give birth.

CHAPTER 1
Continuity of midwifery care

INTRODUCTION

This chapter provides an overview of midwifery continuity of care from three perspectives: a mother, a midwife and a midwifery student. Midwifery continuity of care can be defined as care provided to a woman throughout pregnancy, birth and the early parenting period, from one midwife or a small group of midwives (Sandall et al., 2016). Benefits of midwifery continuity of care include a reduction in obstetric interventions including a reduced need for epidural pain relief, reduced incidence of forceps delivery, episiotomy and caesarean sections (McLachlan et al., 2012; Sandall et al., 2016). Importantly, midwifery continuity of care has been found to reduce the rates of preterm birth by 24% (Sandall et al., 2016). Preterm birth is the leading cause of neonatal death and long-term disability in children (World Health Organization, 2018). A systematic review that evaluated interventions to prevent preterm birth recommended midwifery continuity of care as an effective intervention (Medley et al., 2018). Both women and midwives build a relationship of trust through pregnancy, birth and the early parenting period when they experience midwifery continuity of care. In addition, midwifery continuity of care has been found to be highly satisfying to women and midwives alike.

Women at low risk of medical complications have found midwifery continuity of care increases their satisfaction with antenatal, intrapartum and postpartum care (Forster et al., 2016). An earlier study found women liked the accessibility of midwifery continuity of care; however, this was dependent on the personal and professional attributes of the midwife (Forster et al., 2016). Midwives are less likely to experience work-related burnout as a relationship of trust is built (Newton et al., 2014).

Midwifery continuity of care has been evaluated in low-income settings and found to be satisfying to women (Mortensen, 2019). A scoping review included 175 studies and reports of midwifery continuity of care in high- (157, 90%), middle- to low- (18, 10%) income countries and found no countries have managed to implement and scale up midwifery continuity of care models at a national level, except for New Zealand (Bradford et al., 2022). Further implementation studies are needed to support the transition to midwifery continuity of care in all countries and to determine the optimal model types and strategies to achieve sustainable scale-up at a national level (Bradford et al., 2022). All of this high-level evidence on the benefits of midwifery continuity of care for women, their families and the midwives has informed midwifery education programs.

The International Confederation of Midwives' global standard for midwifery education states students participate in providing midwife-led continuity of care to women/families through pregnancy, birth and the postnatal period (International Confederation of Midwives, 2021). This guidance informs international midwifery curriculums. The Australian midwifery curriculum requires midwifery students to complete 'at least ten continuity of midwifery care experiences' (Australian Nursing and Midwifery Accreditation Council, 2021). Both women and midwifery students value the midwifery continuity of care experiences (Browne & Taylor, 2014; Ferguson et al., 2018; Stulz et al., 2020). Research has found these experiences prepare students to transition to working in midwifery continuity of care at the time of graduation (Cummins et al., 2018). This is most apparent when midwifery students are placed within a midwifery continuity of care model, often called Midwifery Group Practice (MGP) or caseload midwifery (Baird et al., 2021; Carter et al., 2015; Sidebotham & Fenwick, 2019). Preparing students to work in midwifery continuity of care will assist in the scale-up of the models of care so more women have access to this gold standard of maternity care.

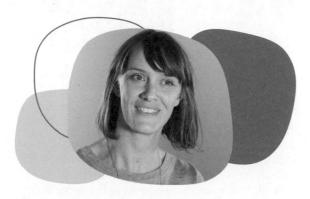

Sarah's story

 View Sarah's story or read the transcript.

Sarah chose midwifery-led continuity of care for her first baby, Isla. She describes how she met a small group of four midwives who provided care to her. Sarah states she mostly saw Christine and felt confident seeing the same midwife who attended the birth of Isla. In addition, Sarah had continuity of care from a midwifery student (Tamara) who was present throughout Sarah's antenatal care and the birth of her daughter. Sarah developed a trusting professional relationship with both the midwife and the student during her pregnancy. She describes how her birth was very intimate with the only people present being her husband, Christine and Tamara.

Sarah describes the midwifery student, Tamara, as being particularly helpful in assisting her to breastfeed immediately at birth. Sarah enjoyed staying in the hospital for a few days in order to receive support with breastfeeding Isla. Sarah continues to tell her story of early mothering.

Reflection

1. Think about how Sarah describes her birth as intimate. What factors contributed to Sarah's intimate birth experience?

2. Sarah discusses how the student midwife was there to support her with breastfeeding straight away. Consider the unique position of midwifery students to support women with initiating breastfeeding as soon as possible after birth.

3. Reflect on Sarah's account of the benefits of staying in hospital in the first few days after Isla's birth.

4. Sarah continues to describe establishing breastfeeding in the first few weeks. Consider some of the challenges women experience when establishing breastfeeding in the first weeks of the baby's life.

Inquiry

1. Read Chapter 1 in *Midwifery Continuity of Care* (2nd ed.) (Homer et al., 2019).
   - Discuss the definitions of midwifery continuity of care and the evidence that supports the benefits of this model of care.

2. Read the article 'Benefits of continuity models of care in building mutual support and nurturing between women and midwifery students. Does continuity of care foster clinical confidence, emotional resilience and influence career goals?' by Ferguson and colleagues (2018).
   - Describe the benefits and challenges midwifery students experience when engaging in midwifery continuity of care experiences.

3. Sarah stated, 'I think I was really lucky, my husband was very helpful. I think he couldn't believe how hard breastfeeding actually could be at the beginning.' Consult the article: 'Women's perceptions and experiences of breastfeeding: A scoping review of the literature' by Beggs and colleagues (2021).
   - Discuss what kind of support is helpful to women in establishing and maintaining breastfeeding.

Action

1. It is proposed that midwifery continuity of care is beneficial for women. Consult the literature on midwifery continuity of care and write a list of the benefits for women and babies.

2. How can women in your local hospital catchment (geographical) area access midwifery continuity of care models?

3. What factors, issues and conditions may exclude the woman from having access to midwifery continuity of care?

4. Discuss the use of the Australian College of Midwives' *National Midwifery Guidelines for Consultation and Referral* (4th ed.) (2021) when providing midwifery continuity of care.

    • Identify a number of reasons that might require consultation and referral to an obstetrician or other practitioner for a woman choosing midwifery-led continuity of care.

5. Discuss how midwifery continuity of care models can be advantageous for women who have complexities in their pregnancy, including women from low socioeconomic circumstances.

Text links

Chapter 1 in *Midwifery Continuity of Care* (2nd ed.). (Homer et al., 2019).

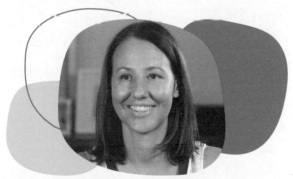

Tamara's story

 View Tamara's story or read the transcript.

Tamara describes how the continuity of care experience helped her learning because she knew the woman. She also describes how the women are keen to assist the student with learning. Tamara experienced one woman confiding in her a very personal traumatic life event because she felt a relationship of trust with Tamara. The relationship with the woman and her family is described by Tamara as one of the best and most positive aspects of her clinical education. In addition, the extra clinical hours that the continuity of care experience provided for Tamara and other midwifery students have been described as highly valuable.

Part of Tamara's story focuses on providing midwifery continuity of care to Sarah alongside a caseload midwife who works in a small midwifery group practice.

Reflection

1. Think about the ways in which continuity of care experiences have helped your learning in the clinical setting.

2. Working with women in a continuity of care experience means that the relationship has the potential for becoming a friendship. Reflect on the differences between friendships and professional relationships. Use the *Australian Nurses and Midwives Board Midwife Standards for Practice*, in relation to standard 2.7: 'develops, maintains and concludes professional relationships in a way that differentiates the boundaries between professional and personal relationships' (Nursing and Midwifery Board of Australia, 2018).

3. Think about some of the feelings you may experience if a woman for whom you have provided continuity of care decides she no longer wants to participate in the program and have you present at her birth.

4. Think about some of the feelings you may experience if a woman for whom you are providing continuity of care experiences a miscarriage or fetal death in utero.

Inquiry

1. How can you enhance your midwifery continuity of care experiences?

2. What factors do you need to consider when on call for a woman's birth?

3. How will you manage your work–life balance?

4. How will you manage the professional boundaries that have the potential to become blurred?

Action

1. Write down a statement that you can use to practise inviting women to participate in the midwifery student continuity of care program.

2. Design and produce a leaflet or pamphlet to offer women when you invite them to participate in the continuity of care experience.

3. Set 10 realistic goals and strategies within a specified time frame for achieving the midwifery continuity of care program. For example, 'Next time I work in the antenatal setting, I will ask a midwife to introduce me to women who may be interested in participating in the continuity of care program'.

4. Write a list of supports (both professional and personal) you can access if you feel that the continuity of care experiences are becoming overwhelming or if you experience a sad event such as one of the women for whom you are providing continuity of care suffers from pregnancy loss.

5. Write a reflective journal of the learning experiences you have gained from continuity of care experiences that you may not have achieved in other clinical settings.

6. In your reflective journal, discuss the scope of practice of a midwifery student in line with the Midwife Standards for Practice point 2.7, mentioned earlier in the chapter.

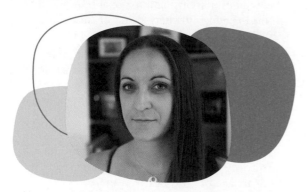

Christine's story

 View Christine's story or read the transcript.

Christine tells her story of how she became a midwife working in a midwifery continuity of care practice. Christine says that her undergraduate midwifery degree prepared her to work in continuity of care. Christine states that working in midwifery continuity of care makes her feel like a 'real midwife'. Part of feeling like a real midwife is working across the full scope of practice with women. Christine states that providing continuity of care to Sarah was a great experience. She also talks about the relationship she has with the women with whom she provides continuity of midwifery care and her small midwifery group practice in a positive manner. Christine also values teaching students as a great part of her work as a midwife.

Reflection

1. Think about how midwifery continuity of care improves midwives' job satisfaction and how it reduces midwives' experiences of job-related stress and burnout.

2. Christine describes the positive relationship she develops with women. Think about how the relationships impact on her professional life.

3. Think about the way you need to work as a midwife providing continuity of midwifery care and the relationships you need to have with your colleagues (including obstetricians) when you work in this way.

4. As described by Christine, working in midwifery continuity of care can be hectic at times. Think about ways you can manage your work–life balance.

Inquiry

1. Research evidence demonstrates that midwifery students are well placed to transition to midwifery continuity of care models at the time of registration. Read the article 'Enabling new graduate midwives to work in midwifery continuity of care models: A conceptual model for implementation' by Cummins and colleagues (2018).

2. How will you prepare to apply for a position in midwifery continuity of care?

Action

1. Develop a checklist of activities to be completed to enable your transition to midwifery continuity of care at the time of graduation.

2. Prepare a goal sheet of the skills you think are necessary to work in continuity of care.

3. If you prefer not to work in continuity of care and are planning to work in one area of midwifery, provide a statement of how you will maintain all your skills to work across the full scope of practice as a midwife.

4. Identify and write down the attributes you need to work in a small team.

5. Prepare an application for a midwifery continuity of care position within two years of graduating. Include in your application the experience you have of continuity of care from your midwifery degree in addition to the skills and attributes you would bring to the position.

Text links

Chapter 17 in *Midwifery: Preparation for Practice* (5th ed.) by Pairman and colleagues (2022).

A FINAL WORD

Sarah, Christine and Tamara talk about their positive experiences of midwifery continuity of care. Sarah's satisfaction with knowing her midwife and having a student midwife with her mirrors the literature of women feeling satisfied with the experience of midwifery continuity of care (Forster et al., 2016). Sarah describes a positive and intimate birth experience with great support in the early mothering period and, in particular, in establishing breastfeeding. Government reports recommend the expansion of publicly funded midwifery-led models of care (COAG Health Council, 2019). Sarah states that she felt quite 'disheartened' with the fragmented model of care she received from the hospital and her general practitioner doctor at the beginning of her pregnancy. Many women are unable to obtain midwifery-led care due to the lack of models. Think about how Australia can expand midwifery-led continuity of care in the public sector so more women like Sarah can access the service.

Midwifery students value the continuity of care experiences that provide an opportunity to develop meaningful, trusting relationships with women. The experiences increase the clinical hours for the midwifery students. As Tamara says, it is easier to learn and practise midwifery skills when you know the woman. Some challenges faced by students during the continuity of care experiences include struggling with the professional boundaries, being on call for births and managing a healthy work–life balance. Midwifery is emotional work and midwifery students and midwives need to manage their emotional connections with women in professional relationships to sustain their career (Catling et al., 2022). Overall, Tamara describes how providing continuity of care as a midwifery student gave her glimpses into becoming a 'real midwife'. Midwifery students are in a unique position to provide midwifery continuity of care and should feel privileged to have the opportunity, despite some of the challenges.

Christine describes being prepared to work in midwifery continuity of care from her degree. New graduate midwives working in midwifery continuity of care within the first year or two of practice have said that they felt prepared to work in continuity of care from their degree and that they felt like a real midwife when working in midwifery continuity of care (Cummins et al., 2015, 2018). Christine reports feeling like a real midwife by keeping her skills up-to-date and not being stuck in only one area of midwifery practice. She is also supported by the team she works alongside. Christine describes the relationship with the women as the best thing about working in continuity of care and the relationship with the small group of midwives as highly satisfying. Christine has a flexible and autonomous way of working in midwifery continuity of care, with great outcomes for the mother and baby.

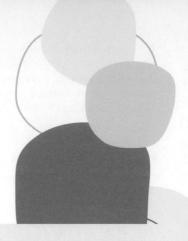

CHAPTER 2
Homebirth

INTRODUCTION

The couple in this chapter, Kaitlin and Scott, describe how they came to choose a homebirth. Kaitlin and Scott had a very positive birth experience with a known midwife; however, the rates of homebirth in Australia are very low: 0.4% of women (927) gave birth at home in 2020 (Australian Institute of Health Welfare, 2022).

Place of birth has been studied in the international and national contexts and found to be safe when the woman is cared for by a qualified midwife networked into the health system (Brocklehurst et al., 2011; Davis et al., 2011; de Jonge et al., 2009; Hutton et al., 2019). In Australia, the odds of women having a normal labour and birth are twice as high in a birth centre and nearly six times as high in planned homebirths, without any significant differences in the proportion of intrapartum stillbirths and early or late neonatal deaths between the hospital, birth centre and home as planned places of birth (Homer et al., 2019). The authors from the place of birth in Australia study concluded that the lower odds of maternal and neonatal complications for women who birth at home compared with those in hospital support the expansion of homebirth options for women without complications in pregnancy.

In Australia there are fewer than 20 publicly funded homebirth services and two states, Queensland and Tasmania, do not offer publicly funded homebirth (Catling, 2020) despite consumer demand for over a decade (Dahlen et al., 2011). Women who are unable to access publicly funded homebirth employ a privately practising midwife.

During the COVID-19 pandemic, over 90% of 103 privately practising midwives surveyed in Australia reported an increase in enquiries for a homebirth (Homer et al., 2021), and the 'Birth in the Time of COVID' study stated that the cost of a midwife with limited rebates through private and public medical insurance in Australia could be seen as a barrier (Kluwgant et al., 2022).

By the end of this chapter, you should be able to identify the facilitators of, and barriers to, women and their partners choosing a homebirth in Australia.

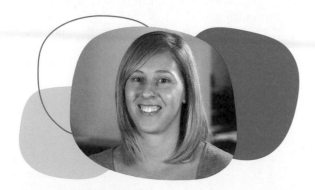

Kaitlin's story

 View Kaitlin's story or read the transcript.

Kaitlin is a woman who chooses a homebirth for the birth of her first baby, Hunter. Kaitlin discusses how she came to the decision to have a homebirth and how she found her midwife. She tells her birth story, including the lead-up to the birth and the day of the labour and birth. Kaitlin also tells us about her experience of early mothering with home visits from her known midwife, Sheryl.

Reflection

1. At the start of her story, Kaitlin discusses the research they did before deciding to have a homebirth. Consider how Australian women decide where they want to give birth and who their care provider will be.

2. Kaitlin chose a privately practising midwife to provide her maternity care. What other options are there for women in Australia to have a homebirth?

3. Support in labour has been reported in the literature to improve outcomes for women and babies (Bohren et al., 2017). Take notice of how Kaitlin describes Scott's role in supporting her in labour.

4. Exclusive breastfeeding is recommended by the WHO (World Health Organization, 2023). Kaitlin attached Hunter at the breast soon after birth. Consider Sheryl's role in assisting Kaitlin to establish breastfeeding.

Inquiry

1. What influenced Kaitlin the most in her decision to have a homebirth?

2. How did Kaitlin and Scott prepare for the homebirth of their baby, Hunter?

3. What strategies did Kaitlin use in the pre-labour phase?

4. What was Kaitlin's main support for labour?

5. Kaitlin discusses what helped her to give birth. Make a list of what helped her.

6. Kaitlin states that giving birth at home was wonderful. Which aspects were wonderful?

7. From Kaitlin's perspective, what was the best thing that Sheryl did in those early days after the birth?

8. How did the midwife, Sheryl, assist Kaitlin to establish breastfeeding?

Action

Find and review the following websites; 'National Publicly Funded Homebirth Consortium' and the 'Find A Midwife' site. Review the National Midwifery Guidelines for Consultation and Referral (Australian College of Midwives, 2021).

A woman approaches you requesting a homebirth. Complete the following actions:
1. Write a brief list of topics you would discuss with the woman.
2. How could this woman access homebirth in your local area?
3. What factors/issues/conditions may exclude the woman from having a homebirth?
4. What will the woman need to do to prepare for a homebirth?
5. What resources/professionals will you (as the midwife) need to access to provide homebirth services?
6. Who will you collaborate with in order to provide a homebirth for the woman?
7. Identify a number of reasons that might require consultation and referral to an obstetrician for a woman choosing a homebirth.
8. What resources would you locate to guide your practice in relation to consultation and referral?

Text links

Chapter 7: 'Birthplace and birth space' in Pairman and colleagues (2022).

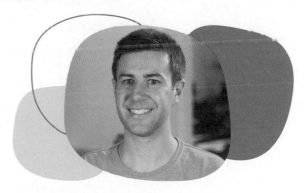

Scott's story

 View Scott's story or read the transcript.

Scott begins by telling us how very happy he is to talk about homebirth. Scott talks about Kaitlin being amazing in labour and birth and how he felt 'she was completely in control'. Scott describes how he did not realise how supportive his actions were to Kaitlin until after the birth and says that the whole birth process was emotional and very positive. Scott also states he was glad when Sheryl arrived for the birth.

Reflection

1. Think about preparing fathers and other support people for a homebirth. What obstacles might fathers experience in their decision-making process?
2. How do fathers view their role during the labour and birth process at home?

Inquiry

1. How did Scott support Kaitlin during her labour and birth?
2. How did Scott view the arrival of Sheryl, the midwife?

Action

Read the following articles and describe how fathers feel about being present at homebirths, particularly when compared with being present at hospital births.

- 'She leads, he follows – fathers' experiences of a planned home birth: A Swedish interview study' by Helena Lindgren and Kerstin Erlandsson (2011).
- 'Put the magic back into life: Fathers' experience of planned home birth' by Siobhan Sweeney and Rhona O'Connell (2015).

A FINAL WORD

Kaitlin and Scott decided to have a homebirth with a privately practising midwife. The story that Kaitlin tells is of a very positive birth experience, with great support from her partner Scott and her midwife. In many developed countries, homebirth with a registered midwife has been shown to be safe for women who are at low risk of obstetric/medical complications, when there are back-up systems of care in place (Brocklehurst et al., 2011; de Jonge et al., 2009; Homer et al., 2019). Think about how Australia can expand its publicly funded homebirth services to make them more available to women like Kaitlin.

CHAPTER 3

Vaginal breech birth

INTRODUCTION

Breech presentation occurs in 3 to 4% of all births (Marshall & Raynor, 2020). Following publication of the international Term Breech Trial (Hannah et al., 2000), the number of vaginal breech births in the developed world plummeted in favour of elective caesarean sections. Currently, most women with a breech baby will give birth by caesarean section, despite the subsequent discrediting of the Term Breech Trial. The optimal mode of birth for women who have a baby in the breech position is the subject of much controversy. However, there is a growing interest in supporting women who choose a vaginal breech birth.

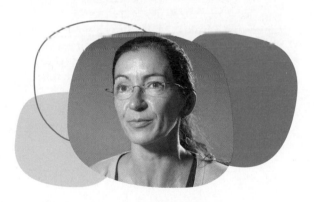

with a breech presentation at 36 weeks' gestation and for midwifery students.

Anke's story

 View Anke's story or read the transcript.

Anke is a German obstetrician who specialises in breech births and maternal/fetal medicine. Listen to Anke's views on the Term Breech Trial, professional development programs for midwives and obstetricians, and external cephalic version (ECV). She also shares some valuable advice for a woman who is diagnosed

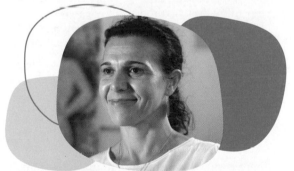

Karolina's story

 View Karolina's story or read the transcript.

Karolina is a mother of two children who had a vaginal breech birth with her second baby. Karolina experienced a very straightforward vaginal breech birth but

the period from 36 weeks' gestation leading up to the birth was fraught with anxiety and stress. Listening to her story, you will hear Karolina describe social isolation and challenging situations. While this is disappointing, Karolina's story can teach us about the ways midwives can positively support women and their partners when their baby is in the breech position.

Reflection

1. Karolina talks about the difficulties she experienced trying to access quality information on vaginal breech birth. What information did Karolina find 'powerful' when deciding to have a vaginal breech birth?

2. Explain why you think a woman has the right to make an informed choice whether or not to have a vaginal breech birth.

3. Karolina's experience of labour was very positive. What did the midwives and obstetricians do to 'normalise' Karolina's birth?

4. Karolina offers advice for midwives and midwifery students. How will you, as the midwife, support a woman's choice regarding her mode of birth when her baby is in the breech presentation?

Inquiry

1. An external cephalic version (ECV) is a useful technique to 'turn a breech' and has been practised since the time of Hippocrates. Consult your midwifery textbook and research the indications, criteria, contraindications and procedure for ECV.

2. In Australia, breech birth is considered to fall outside the scope of the midwife's practice.

However, the Nursing and Midwifery Board of Australia's Midwife Standards for Practice (2018) expect midwives to 'recognise and respond effectively in emergency or urgent situations'. Sometimes a breech presentation is unexpectedly diagnosed in labour. Consult your midwifery textbook on the mechanism of breech labour and the technique of birthing a breech baby.

Action

1. The Term Breech Trial has been criticised on methodological grounds, thereby making its applicability to well-resourced Australian and New Zealand hospitals uncertain. Locate the Royal Australian and New Zealand College of Obstetricians and Gynaecologists (RANZCOG) College Statement (2016) on Management of Breech Presentation at Term and read it critically.

2. It is critical that clinicians who work in maternity care settings are able to support and care for women who have a breech baby. Becoming a Breech Expert (BABE©) is an ALSO (Advanced Life Support in Obstetrics) Course. Currently, it is a one-day course that takes participants on a journey with a woman who has a breech baby and wants to have a vaginal birth. The aim of the BABE© Course is to provide participants with the knowledge of the key practical issues in supporting a woman with a breech presentation and, in particular, the skills in managing a vaginal breech birth. Find out where the nearest course is being held and consider attending. Share this information with your colleagues.

3. Speak to some experienced midwives and ask them what experience they have of assisting women to give birth to breech babies.

A FINAL WORD

There is much controversy around the optimal mode of birth for women who have a baby in the breech position. It is important to remember that unexpected breech birth continues to occur, particularly in women having a preterm labour and birth. Therefore, it is critical that clinicians who work in maternity care settings are trained to be able to competently support and care for women who are having a vaginal breech birth.

CHAPTER 4

Having a baby over 40 years of age

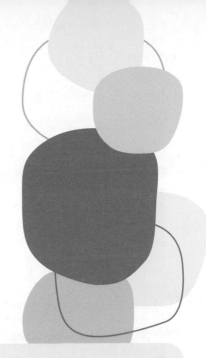

INTRODUCTION

Having a baby later in life can mean that some women have greater health challenges to face. The number of women who choose to delay childbearing has increased greatly in recent years, prompting consideration of the social, political, environmental and lifestyle factors contributing to the trend (Aitken, 2022). Delaying pregnancy is also associated with an increase in pregnancy complications and negative maternal and neonatal outcomes. This is in part due to the increased risk of infertility for women over 35 years of age (Seshadri et al., 2021) and the growing reliance on assisted reproduction technology. The success rates of in vitro fertilisation (IVF) fall after 40 years of age with more than 50% of cycles of IVF unsuccessful (Seshadri et al., 2021), meaning delaying pregnancy is often an intensely emotional journey. However, risks are not just confined to women. Studies have also suggested that babies of fathers that delay paternity can also have an increase in genetic disorders (Charalambous et al., 2023).

Despite these challenges, having a baby over 40 is often welcomed as a profoundly joyful time, especially after an emotional journey of miscarriage and fertility treatments.

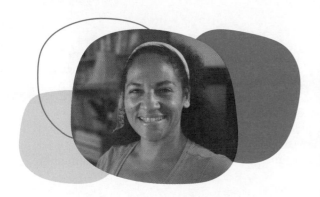

Malika's story

 View Malika's story or read the transcript.

In section 1, Malika discusses her experience of having a baby after 40 years of age. Malika did not have any antenatal complications; however, her baby (Jesse) was treated for sepsis in the early postnatal period. In sections 2 and 3 of the video, Malika talks about her maternity care and the birth of her baby boy, Jesse.

Reflection

1. What do you think are the physical and emotional considerations of having a baby in your 40s?

2. Malika states that she had no problems 'getting back to my body shape' and that she learnt from her previous experiences in her 20s. What advice do you give to women about their general health and weight in the postnatal period?

3. There is a real need to inform prospective parents about the decline in fertility, risk of genetic disorders and rise of perinatal complications with increasing age. Think about how you would discuss these topics with couples.

4. Malika describes the antenatal clinic she attended as 'always running late' and 'in-out-in-out'. How do you think this impacted on Malika's care?

5. When thinking about communication, what are the benefits for the same small team of midwives to care for the same group of women in the antenatal period? See Chapter 1 'Continuity of midwifery care'.

Inquiry

1. Malika's partner wanted her to have extra tests, which she declined. Why would extra antenatal tests be recommended, and what are they?

2. Look in your workplace to see if there is a policy in relation to caring for women over 40 years of age having babies. This information may be located in the antenatal clinic.

3. If possible, talk to the genetic counsellor in your workplace about their antenatal recommendations for older women having a baby.

Action

1. There are several risks of delaying childbearing. Investigate two (2) of the following risks and look at the Clinical Practice Guidelines (Australian Government, Department of Health and Aged Care, 2020) to understand the evidence-based recommendations that should be incorporated into the care of these women:
   - spontaneous abortion
   - ectopic pregnancy
   - placenta praevia
   - gestational diabetes
   - preeclampsia
   - hypertension
   - caesarean section
   - induction of labour
   - chromosomal disorders
   - preterm birth
   - perinatal death.

2. Investigate what services or supports are available to women who experience pregnancy in their 40s. What other factors may be present in women having a baby over the age of 40 years that increase her likelihood of having some of the complications listed above?

A FINAL WORD

In recent years, the proportion of women over the age of 35 who have babies has increased significantly. This is associated with an increased risk of complications (some listed in Action question 1). Most women would be aware of their 'biological clock' and accept that there may be more difficulties in pregnancy and birth associated with age. Some women, like Malika, will have few problems. However, it is necessary to ensure that women who delay childbearing are counselled appropriately and given information about these risks. In addition, women need to be appropriately informed about the extra antenatal testing that is offered, and their decisions to either go ahead with testing, or not, should be respected.

CHAPTER 5

Grand multiparity

INTRODUCTION

Being classified as a 'grand multiparous' woman will vary depending on the literature. Some define grand-multiparity as equal to or greater than five births at a gestation of 20 weeks or more, while others will suggest it is greater than four or greater than six births. The term 'great grand multiparity' is given to a woman who has had 10 or more births (Muniro et al., 2019). In high-resource countries such as Australia, grand multiparity accounts for only 3 to 4% of all births, whereas in low-resource countries with lower access to contraception, it is relatively common.

The traditional view of grand multiparous women has been that they had more complicated births, poorer maternal and neonatal outcomes, and in particular were at a higher risk of postpartum haemorrhage. Grand multiparous women can have more complications during their pregnancies and birth due to many other factors (not just their parity) (Al-Shaikh et al., 2017). For example, they may have had smaller inter-pregnancy intervals that predispose them to anaemia. Also, independent of how many babies they have had, the women may be over the age of 40, which predisposes them to other pregnancy complications including fetal chromosomal abnormalities. This is discussed in a large cohort study by Hochler and colleagues (2020).

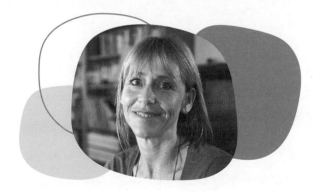

Emma is a woman who has given birth to seven children. She discusses how she was cared for and how she felt about having her babies (section 1), her psychological preparation for birth (section 2) and the midwifery care she had that was effective—and not so effective (section 3). Emma also discusses the social side of having a large family (section 4).

Reflection

Emma was told she might be at a higher risk of bleeding after birth and that her contractions may not be effective. She was not particularly concerned about this and had great faith in her body's ability to give birth.

1. Emma describes her post-baby body as showing the 'story of my life'. Think about how you can help women accept their body's changes after childbirth.

Emma's story

 View Emma's story or read the transcript.

2. Psychological preparation for having a baby is necessary for all women. Think about what this actually means. Why do you think being mentally prepared for labour and birth is necessary?

3. How could psychological preparation for birth be facilitated? Think about how you would do this when caring for a woman at term.

4. Emma explains the good qualities she found in some of the midwives who cared for her. Think of a time when you witnessed such care, and how it may have made the woman feel.

5. Have you had somebody listen to you when you are telling them something important (but not *really* listen)? How did that make you feel?

Inquiry

1. Confidence and attitude to pregnancy and birth are important in relation to how women feel and cope in the postnatal period. Read the *Code of Conduct for Midwives* at https://www.nursingmidwiferyboard.gov.au/codes-guidelines-statements/professional-standards.aspx

2. Which explanatory point covers how midwives need to support and engender women's confidence?

3. Check your workplace to find out if there is a local policy on the care of grand multiparous women. If so, how does it differ to caring for other women in labour?

4. Research grand multiparity and postpartum haemorrhage (PPH). Report the findings.

5. List the words that Emma uses to describe midwives. One word that is used more than once is the concept of 'kindness' in midwives. Research 'intelligent kindness' and find out what this means.

6. Listen and watch other midwives you work with. What non-verbal behaviour do they display that women may describe as 'kind'?

7. Approach a social worker in your workplace and find out what support is available for women with five or more children.

Action

1. Ensure you are familiar with your local policy of caring for grand multiparous women.

2. Look at the Australian College of Midwives' National Midwifery Guidelines for Consultation and Referral. What category does grand multiparity come under? What does this mean?

3. Have a personal 'toolkit' of questions and information to share with women to help them mentally prepare for birth in their third trimester.

4. Research 'effective listening skills' and find out what it means to probe, reflect, deflect and advise within conversations. Practise listening effectively to a colleague. Begin the conversation by saying, 'Did you have a nice weekend?' and then probe and reflect to find out more.

5. Emma has put her career 'on hold' since she became a mother. Gain a clear idea of maternity and paternity leave entitlements in Australia by exploring the following website: http://www.fairwork.gov.au/Leave/maternity-and-parental-leave.

A FINAL WORD

Having seven children comes with the need/desire to have a larger house, car and income! However, family and community support is also vital for the wellbeing of the mother and her children. During pregnancy and birth, grand multiparous women may have a greater likelihood of complications, but they also have high rates of normal birth.

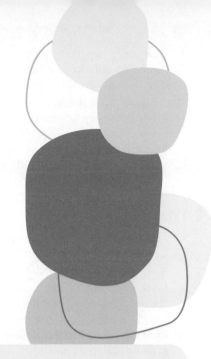

CHAPTER 6

Rural and remote midwifery

INTRODUCTION

Rural and remote midwifery and maternity services in Australia are quite different from those in urban areas. About 7 million people, or 28% of Australians, live in remote and rural areas (AIHW, 2022). Women living in rural and remote Australia have fewer options for care and services than those living in major cities. This means that they often have to relocate to cities to give birth, which can lead to a number of social and financial issues.

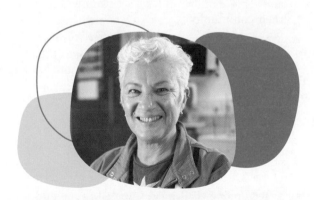

Jane's story

 View Jane's story or read the transcript.

In this video, Jane explains the issues women have in remote settings (sections 1 and 2). In sections 3 and 4, Jane describes her work as a midwife in a remote setting, and in section 5, she explains the importance of birth within the community.

Reflection

1. Reflect on how Jane describes rural and remote women's priorities in relation to their pregnancy and birth.

2. Imagine you have to transfer to a hospital that is 500 km away from your friends and family to await labour and birth. How would your family cope with your absence for what could be around 4 to 6 weeks? In this situation, would you be more inclined to accept an offer of an induction of labour? Imagine how you would feel if you were a woman giving birth without the support of your partner and wider family.

3. What did Jane find good and what was challenging about being a midwife in remote Australia?

4. Jane states that there were problems related to not being able to give continuity of midwifery care. What were these problems?

5. Imagine how the woman felt when she gave birth to a very preterm baby (in Jane's story). Contrast the feelings she may have had giving birth in hospital with those she may have had giving birth within her community.

Inquiry

1. Look up the rate of caesarean section operations in rural and remote Australia. Does this differ markedly from the rate in urban Australia?

2. Look at the latest data from the AIHW's *Australia's Mothers and Babies: Maternal Deaths* (2021) report: https://www.aihw.gov.au/reports/mothers-babies/maternal-deaths-australia. Are rates of maternal death higher in rural and remote areas? What are the factors related to this?

3. Thinking about the demographics of the communities in rural and remote Australia, why do you think Jane saw a lot of growth-restricted babies?

4. What are the rates of antenatal care attendance in women living in rural and remote Australia? What are the factors related to this?

5. Jane discusses practices within hospitals that she suggests were not concurrent with best practice. Look up guidelines that state:
   a. the ideal timing of giving intrapartum pethidine (or morphine) for pain relief
   b. indications for electronic fetal monitoring.

6. Look up the financial assistance women can apply for when they need to transfer to hospital from a remote or rural area to give birth.

7. Locate the national strategy document on *Woman-centred care: Strategic directions for Australian maternity services* (2019): https://www.health.gov.au/resources/publications/woman-centred-care-strategic-directions-for-australian-maternity-services. Consider how the four values and principles of safety, respect, choice and access are impacted for women accessing maternity services in rural and remote settings in Australia.

Action

1. Ensure you have an understanding of the issues rural and remote women face in relation to their pregnancy, birth and postnatal care.

2. Explain how you think these issues could be overcome. For example, could caseload continuity of midwifery care operate in rural and remote areas?

3. Ensure you have an appreciation of the difficulties midwives face when working within rural and remote communities.

4. Find out the availability of continuing professional development activities that rural and remote midwives have access to within their community.

5. Watch the fascinating documentary *Birth Rites* (available through your university library) that compares Canadian and rural and remote Australian maternity services.

A FINAL WORD

Women and their families in rural and remote Australia face unique challenges. Over 100 rural and remote maternity units have been closed in recent years, exacerbating the lack of antenatal and birth services for women and the families who live in these areas. Rather than focusing on a family-oriented birth, women in these areas are often more preoccupied with the practicalities of where and when they will give birth. As outlined in this chapter, this is often within a hospital many kilometres away from home; consequently, sometimes women have no family accompanying them. It is important, as a midwife, to acknowledge the challenges women have to face when living in a rural and remote area.

CHAPTER 7

Caesarean section

INTRODUCTION

This chapter introduces you to women experiencing caesarean section. There are stories from two women. The first is Melanie, a woman who chooses to have a caesarean section, and the second woman is Katie, who undergoes an emergency caesarean section. For over a century, access to and increased safety of caesarean sections has played an important part in improving outcomes for mothers and babies who experience this intervention. There are several medical indications for caesarean section including antepartum haemorrhage, cord prolapse, eclampsia, uterine rupture, labour dystocia and fetal distress; however, there is concern that there has been a general increase in caesarean section for non-medical reasons.

The *Australia's Mothers and Babies* report (AIHW, 2021), states that one in three mothers gave birth by caesarean section in 2020. The rate of women giving birth by caesarean section has risen from 32% in 2010 to 37% in 2020. There is also a significant difference between private and public hospital rates, 49.9% (private) versus 35% (public) (AIHW, 2021). The steep rise in caesarean section rates is likely to be due to a number of maternal, clinical and medico-legal factors, but the reasons behind the increase remain largely unknown (AIHW, 2021; Betran et al., 2016).

The World Health Organization (WHO) recommends several non-clinical interventions to reduce unnecessary caesarean sections (WHO, 2018). Interventions to reduce caesarean section births include the use of evidence-based clinical practice guidelines with a mandatory second opinion for caesarean section indication and caesarean section audits with well-timed feedback to healthcare professionals (WHO, 2018). The midwifery code of professional conduct for midwives in Australia states that midwives should promote normal birth (NMBA, 2018). Furthermore, research recommends the implementation of midwifery-led models of care as an intervention to decrease caesarean section rates (Hanahoe, 2020). It is widely accepted across maternity care services in Australia that every decision regarding whether to perform a caesarean section or not is discussed with the woman and clinicians must inform her about both the short- and the long-term risks and the benefits of the operation, whether it is an elective or an unplanned emergency procedure.

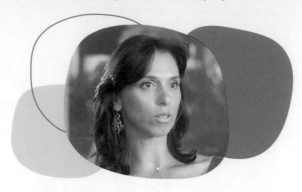

Melanie's story: an elective caesarean section

 View Melanie's story or read the transcript.

Melanie chose an elective caesarean section for her first baby, Jake. She is currently pregnant with her second baby and plans a caesarean section again. In Australia, 32.9% of babies were born via caesarean section in 2011. Melanie discusses how she came to the decision to have an elective caesarean section and how she found a private obstetrician who would offer an elective caesarean section. Melanie tells her birth story, including the lead-up to the birth and the day of the operation. Melanie also tells us about her experience of early mothering in a private hospital with discharge to a hotel as part of the private hospital package.

Reflection

1. In the first part of the video, Melanie discusses how she read a lot of information about caesarean sections and was influenced by her relatives who are doctors. Consider how Australian women decide where to give birth, by what mode (vaginal or caesarean) and who their care provider will be.

2. Melanie chose a privately practising obstetrician to provide her maternity care. What other options are there for women in Australia to have an elective caesarean?

3. Complications from caesarean sections include increased blood loss, decreased mobility for the mother and increased need for pain-relieving drugs in the early parenting period. Consider how Melanie managed these associated complications.

4. Early breastfeeding is recommended by the World Health Organization. Melanie was able to perform skin-to-skin contact in the operating theatre. Think about how this may have helped Melanie to initiate and maintain breastfeeding.

Inquiry

1. What influenced Melanie the most in her decision to have an elective caesarean section?

2. How did Melanie prepare for the caesarean birth of her baby, Jake?

3. What was helpful to Melanie when she was about to undergo surgery?

4. What surprised Melanie about the people present at her birth?

5. What was helpful to Melanie during the operation?

6. How did Melanie see her role in the birth of Jake?

7. What do you think Melanie means when she states 'you're in the hands of the professionals'?

8. From Melanie's perspective, what was important to her at the birth?

9. How did Melanie describe the support she received in the initial postnatal period, when she returned to her room following the caesarean?

10. Melanie talks about receiving conflicting advice from the midwives in the early parenting period. The best thing for Melanie was having a lactation consultant come and visit her in hospital and at home. Consider what support the lactation consultant provided Melanie, including the language the consultant used.

Action

A woman approaches you requesting an elective cae-sarean because she is very frightened about giving birth 'naturally' (vaginally). Consult the resources provided and complete the following.

1. Write a brief list of topics you would discuss with the woman.

2. What resources/professionals will you (as the midwife) need to access to provide a

comprehensive discussion about elective caesarean section?

3. Discuss the implications for the woman's recovery post-caesarean section.

4. Discuss the implications for the woman's next pregnancy.

5. Discuss the implications for the baby.

6. What resources would you source to guide your practice in relation to consultation and referral?

Text links

Chapter 39 'Interventions in pregnancy, labour and birth', *Midwifery: Preparation for Practice* (Pairman et al., 2022).

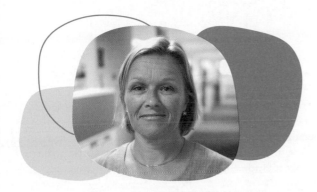

Katie's story: emergency caesarean birth

 View Katie's story or read the transcript.

Katie's first baby was born via emergency caesarean section due to fetal distress. Katie shares her insight about the ways that midwives can better support women undergoing an emergency caesarean section.

Reflection

1. Katie talks about the very short time interval from the decision to deliver by caesarean section to the actual birth of her baby. Reflect on some strategies that you can develop to involve women and their partners in the decision-making process, even in an emergency situation.

2. Katie valued having been part of a team midwifery model of care. Reflect on the positive impact of continuity of midwifery care, particularly during and following an emergency caesarean section.

3. Katie considers the postnatal care she received following her emergency caesarean birth. She expresses the need for clear guidance or information to be given to the mother on what to expect postnatally. Reflect on some approaches that you can take to address this issue.

4. Women can be deeply scarred by traumatic birthing. Reflect on some strategies that you can develop to minimise the emotional trauma.

Inquiry

1. Consult a current midwifery textbook (e.g. *Myles Textbook for Midwives*, 17th ed., 2020) and research caesarean section (e.g. preparation, anaesthesia, postoperative care, postnatal care and complications associated with caesarean section).

2. Familiarise yourself with the Australian College of Midwives' *National Midwifery Guidelines for Consultation and Referral* (2021). These guidelines are for midwives and help to ensure that the midwifery care they provide to women and babies is high quality, safe and collaborative. Guideline 8.1.4 Clinical indications during labour and birth is specific to conditions or abnormalities that are identified during labour and birth, which may result in an emergency caesarean section.

3. Read the article by Mapp and Hudson (2005) on feelings and fears during obstetric emergencies. Consider some of the strategies that the authors provide aimed at 'minimising' the emotional trauma of an emergency caesarean section and endeavour to incorporate these into your everyday clinical practice.

4. If the indication for caesarean has been a non-recurring one (e.g. fetal distress), vaginal birth after caesarean (VBAC) may be attempted. Read Trish's story in Chapter 14.

5. Visit the Raising Children website (https://raisingchildren.net.au/pregnancy/labour-birth/recovery-after-birth/after-caesarean). The resources on this website include: going home after caesarean birth, feelings after caesarean birth; bleeding after caesarean; pain relief after caesarean; caesarean wound care; practical help after caesarean; exercise, food and sleep after

caesarean; relationships and friendships after birth; breastfeeding after caesarean; and the 6-week check.

Action

1. Revise and keep your emergency skills and knowledge up to date (e.g. maternal and neonatal resuscitation).

2. Some women may have a lingering feeling of failure or disappointment at having had an emergency caesarean section and may value the opportunity to talk this over with a midwife or clinician. Women who have had a caesarean section should be offered an opportunity to discuss the reasons and be given written information about their caesarean section and birth options for future pregnancies (NSW Health, 2010).

3. Read the article by Mapp and Hudson 2005b (Part 2) on the importance of debriefing after a traumatic obstetric emergency such as an emergency caesarean section.

4. Find out if following their first caesarean section, women in your hospital get clear information (both verbally and printed) about birth options for any future pregnancies.

5. Download the NSW Health Guideline, *Maternity—Supporting Women in Their Next Birth After Caesarean Section* (2014) so that you are aware of the guideline and actively participate in its implementation to support pregnant women who have had a previous caesarean section in their decision making around their next birth after caesarean section (NBAC).

A FINAL WORD

As the caesarean section rate continues to increase, women like Melanie and Katie need to be made aware of the benefits and the risks associated with the surgery. As a midwife, you are in a good position to offer the information to the woman and her partner. The information needs to be conveyed in a non-judgemental manner at the earliest possible time in the woman's pregnancy or during the preconception period. The information should not only include the expected outcomes for this pregnancy, but also for future planned or unplanned pregnancies.

CHAPTER 8

Same-sex parenting

INTRODUCTION

In the 2016 Census, Australia was reported to have over 46,800 same-sex couples, which was a 39% increase from the 2011 Census. This comprises 23,300 male same-sex couples and 23,000 female same-sex couples (ABS, 2018). Only one in a thousand of all children are from same-sex couples, and 15% of all same-sex partnerships include at least one child. The overwhelming majority of these children had female parents (85%).

Since 2008, through the passing of the Government's same-sex law reform package, same-sex couples and their families no longer experience discrimination in areas such as taxation, superannuation, family assistance and social security, shared expenses on the Pharmaceutical Benefits Scheme and Medicare Safety Net schemes, and child support and family law (Department of Social Services, 2020). Social acceptance and recognition of same-sex partnerships has also increased since the update to the Marriage Act 1961 in 2017 to allow same-sex marriage in Australia. Despite these social and economic improvements, people in same-sex partnerships often still face discrimination, judgement and/or stigma when accessing healthcare services, and this includes maternity care (Sung Soled et al., 2022).

Much ignorance and assumption surrounds attitudes towards same-sex couples, and fear regarding the welfare of children raised in these families. One recent longitudinal study from the Netherlands, the first country to legalise same-sex marriage, found that 'children raised by same-sex parents from birth perform better than children raised by different-sex parents in both primary and secondary education' (Mazrekaj et al., 2020, p. 830). Additionally, a study from Melbourne found that children of same-sex couples scored higher than the national average for overall health and family cohesion (measuring how well a family gets along), although adolescents were negatively affected by external societal stigma (Crouch et al., 2014a). The children also had higher scores on measures of general behaviour compared with children in standard population data (Crouch et al., 2014b; Mazrekaj et al., 2022).

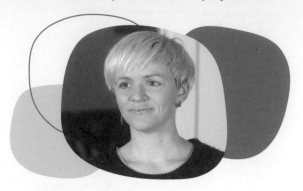

Leia's story

 View Leia's story or read the transcript.

Leia and her partner Toby have a one-year-old girl, Taj. Leia was fortunate to have her own mother, a midwife, care for her throughout her pregnancy, birth and the postnatal period. Listen to Leia's story where she describes sensitive midwifery care (section 1), discriminatory behaviour towards same-sex couples (section 2) and her story of pregnancy (section 3).

Reflection

1. Whenever female same-sex couples attend maternity services, staff need to display non-discriminatory, sensitive care that does not unnecessarily probe into the personal life of the couple. In section 1, Leia describes how some couples can be sensitive to midwives being too inquisitive. What are the pertinent things to know regarding pregnancy/relationships when booking a couple at the first antenatal visit? What aspects do not need to be explored?

2. When meeting a woman for the first time, using the word 'husband' assumes that the woman is married and her partner is male. When using the description 'partner', you may then use 'he' in your language. Before you know the gender of the partner, think about how you can subtly change your language at this first meeting.

3. Read the article by Stewart and O'Reilly (2017). In this article, the attitudes, knowledge and beliefs of nurses and midwives are explored in relation to the healthcare needs of those in the LGBTQ population. Reflect on the models

of care you work in and how they may prompt, or not prompt, couples to comfortably disclose that they are in a same-sex partnership. In what ways can you foster a trusting therapeutic relationship to accommodate the needs of the couple throughout their time accessing maternity care services? It is important to note that some people will feel safer and more comfortable if their lesbian/gay relationship is not known, whereas others may only feel genuine through disclosure.

Inquiry

1. When born to opposite-sex couples, a child will usually have a birth mother and father and both will be legal parents. In same-sex couples, the birth mother is the legal parent under the current family law system, but a lesbian co-mother or gay co-father(s) is not recognised in the same way. Read the current legalities at https://www.humanrights.gov.au/publications/same-sex-same-entitlements-chapter-5#2 and find out what couples should do so that the partner of the birth parent is legally recognised.

2. Midwives need to practise without discrimination and develop respectful partnerships for the women and families in their care. Which standard/s in the Midwife Standards for Practice (Nursing and Midwifery Board of Australia, 2018) discuss respectful partnerships and practising without discrimination?

3. Have a look at this article by Hammond (2014) on same-sex couples' experiences of maternity care: https://www.britishjournalofmidwifery.com/content/research/exploring-same-sex-couples-experiences-of-maternity-care. Why is it so essential for midwives to be educated on the unique needs of lesbian women and gay men when it comes to maternity care?

Action

1. Examine the booking forms and other documentation in your workplace. How could you make your workplace more responsive and aware of lesbian/gay parents through altering data-collection documentation?

2. Put together a factsheet with information for midwives about different family structures, including same-sex parents.

3. In section 2, Leia describes some disturbing discriminatory behaviour directed at herself and her partner. A 'prejudice' is an opinion or attitude about a group of people or individuals, whereas 'discrimination' is behaviour that treats people unequally because of the group to which they belong. Use the internet to find information and tools to examine your own background and beliefs.

A FINAL WORD

Midwives can enhance the experience of same-sex couples who have to negotiate the maternity system by building their own skills and knowledge about the issues these families face. Leia sums it up well by saying, 'It shouldn't make a difference if a couple is a same-sex couple or a heterosexual couple. At the end of the day, it's people having babies.'

CHAPTER 9
Young mothers

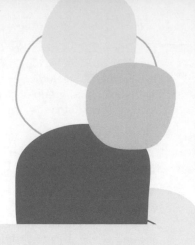

INTRODUCTION

In Australia, the overall proportion of teenage mothers (aged younger than 20) was 2.2% in 2017 (AIHW, 2022), which is lower than in previous years. In developing countries globally, complications during pregnancy and birth form the second-highest cause of death for young women, and remain a major contributor to maternal and infant mortality.

Young women can face particular issues during their pregnancies, birth and the postnatal period. These include higher rates of anaemia (Pinho-Pompeu et al., 2017); preterm birth, low birthweight babies, congenital abnormalities and perinatal death (Karai et al., 2019); and social, emotional and financial difficulties. Young women who are disadvantaged and unsupported may perpetuate a cycle of social disadvantage, poverty and possibly substance abuse (especially smoking). For their infants, this can mean poorer development, ill health and behavioural problems.

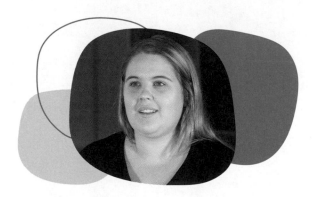

Jordan's story

 View Jordan's story or read the transcript.

In Jordan's story, she describes her first birth experience at age 16 and her second at age 19. With no health complications and a supportive partner and family, Jordan discusses the support she had (sections 1 to 3) and the midwifery care she experienced (section 4).

Reflection

1. Jordan describes quite different experiences between her first and second births. What made them different?

2. Teenage mothers may have a level of emotional immaturity simply because of their age. Think about how midwives can support young women emotionally. Who else could help?

3. Jordan had a thirst for knowledge during her first pregnancy. She describes care from some midwives who 'would talk through everything', which she appreciated. How could continuity of midwifery care be beneficial for young pregnant women?

4. There is social stigma surrounding young parenthood (Mohammed Arshadh & Tengku Muda, 2020). Hence, young mothers and fathers tend to respond more positively to those who are non-judgemental and have

non-authoritarian teaching styles (Nolan & Hendricks, 2019). In your practice, how do you remain non-judgemental?

Inquiry

1. Look at the website https://aifs.gov.au/resources/practice-guides/supporting-young-parents and list the negative and positive implications of teenage pregnancy.

2. Some of the psychosocial risks of childbirth for young women may include: an inability to complete education or secure employment; an inability to maintain friendships or good relations with her partner; and having a feeling of shame associated with being a young mother. Which of these did Jordan experience?

3. The mothers' group Jordan attended consisted of women who were considerably older than her. What ante/postnatal groups are available to teenage mothers in your area?

4. Jordan ceased to breastfeed immediately upon returning home from the birth of her first child, and while in hospital 'felt really judged' and 'traumatised' as though she was 'doing it wrong'. What management plan could have been put in place to help Jordan continue breastfeeding her baby?

5. Does being a teenage mother increase the risks of adverse outcomes for the mother and baby? Research this issue and list the main risks you find. What is the optimal age for pregnancy and childbirth?

Action

1. Think about the complex needs of younger women. Does your workplace provide support for young parents? Are the services sensitive to the needs of young people?

2. Jordan discusses feeling that health practitioners 'pigeon-holed' her as a teenage mother. Nolan and Hendricks (2019) describe that young parents want to be treated like an equal and not told what to do. In your midwifery practice, ensure you treat women as individuals while being mindful of the particular issues that might arise in relation to their circumstances.

A FINAL WORD

Young teenage pregnant women need particular care and support in the perinatal period. Many health districts have specific models of care tailored to the needs of young parents. The role of midwives when caring for teenage mothers is to practise in a non-discriminatory way, focus on her particular needs and promote a trusting relationship to ensure her physical, psychological, emotional and social wellbeing.

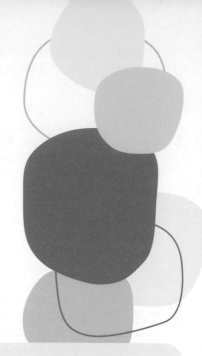

CHAPTER 10

Indigenous mothers and midwives

INTRODUCTION

Improving the health status of Indigenous people in Australia is a longstanding challenge for governments in Australia. The gap in health status between Indigenous and non-Indigenous Australians remains unacceptably wide (AIHW, 2022). In Australia, various health strategies have identified the urgent need to address the disparity between health outcomes of Indigenous people and those of the non-Indigenous population (AIHW, 2022). There is an immediate need for culturally sensitive healthcare to significantly improve the health status of Indigenous people. In keeping with the Nursing and Midwifery Board of Australia's Midwife Standards for Practice (2018) and International Confederation of Midwives Code of Ethics for Midwives (2014), midwives are expected to practise in a culturally sensitive and appropriate manner at all times.

A culturally competent workforce is recognised as a priority reform area in closing the gap in Indigenous life outcomes (Commonwealth of Australia, 2022). The development of organisational, systemic and individual cultural competence is essential to ensure that all Aboriginal and Torres Strait Islander peoples using a health service are treated in a respectful and safe manner that secures their trust in the capacity of the service to meet their needs (Bainbridge et al., 2015). Gaining an understanding of and respect for Indigenous people will enable all healthcare staff (including midwives) to develop meaningful and respectful professional relationships, culminating in improved healthcare outcomes.

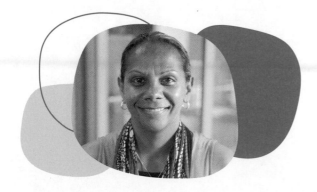

Leona's story

 View Leona's story or read the transcript.

Leona is a very proud Aboriginal woman, a midwife, mother to three children and a grandmother to one boy. Her great-grandmother's people are the Woppaburra people from Great Keppel Island and her great-grandmother was one of the last Aboriginal people taken off this island. Her grandfather is from the Kuku Yalanji people in Far North Queensland. Leona lives in Sydney. She talks about her experiences of pregnancy and birth and her views on Aboriginal midwives and health workers.

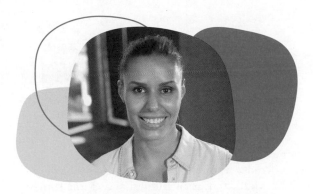

Kate's story

View Kate's story or read the transcript.

Kate is a Wiradjuri woman on her father's side and is a registered midwife. Kate chose midwifery as a career because she wanted to make a difference to her community. She has worked in the Malabar Community Midwifery Service in Sydney for over six years.

Reflection

1. Leona and Kate talk about the importance of having a culturally appropriate community midwifery service. Reflect on the value of having such a service and what you feel is important for engaging with people's cultural identity.

2. Listen to the aspects of Kate's work that she finds most rewarding and notice the benefits of continuity of midwifery care.

3. Listen to the advice that Leona and Kate offer to midwives and midwifery students about providing culturally appropriate care and reflect on the possible implications of this for your developing midwifery practice.

Inquiry

One of the core principles of woman-centred care is that care is holistic in terms of addressing the woman's social, emotional, physical, psychological, spiritual and cultural needs and expectations (NMBA, 2018).

1. Download and read *Cultural competency in the delivery of health services for Indigenous people* (Bainbridge et al., 2015). Identify four principles and strategies for developing culturally competent services.

2. Cultural safety is underpinned by communication and recognition of the diversity in worldviews (both within and between cultural groups). Kate says that midwives should not be afraid to have a conversation with women, and ask if unsure about a woman's cultural needs because engaging with clients helps to break down cultural barriers. In your approach to midwifery care, consider how you can create a climate of cultural safety.

Action

Midwives have an opportunity to make a difference to the lives of women, particularly those women who may already experience disadvantage. As a practising midwife, keep yourself up to date on cultural issues in order to always work in a culturally intelligent and sensitive manner. Here are some examples.

1. Enrol in a cultural education program in your health service to ensure that you are well informed about the health needs of Aboriginal and Torres Strait Islander peoples and the broader determinants of health.

2. Evaluate your personal/professional practice and consider how to construct a workable philosophy of woman-centred care that will make a difference to the provision and delivery of culturally sensitive care.

A FINAL WORD

Aboriginal and Torres Strait Islander women and babies continue to experience higher rates of mortality and morbidity compared with non-Indigenous women and babies. Understanding the unique needs of Aboriginal and Torres Strait Islander families specific to the area of childbirth is an important component of effective and culturally competent care. All practising midwives should keep up to date on cultural issues in order to always work in a culturally intelligent and sensitive manner.

CHAPTER 11
Fathers

INTRODUCTION

The role of the father has changed dramatically in recent decades. Father–child relationships—be they positive, negative or lacking, at any stage in the life of the child, and in all cultural and ethnic communities—have profound and wide-ranging impacts on children that last a lifetime. The benefits of having a father involved in raising his children have become more evident over the past few decades. High levels of father involvement are associated with positive outcomes for children, including better physical and mental health (Allport et al., 2018), and can have a positive effect on future generations (Jessee & Adamsons, 2018).

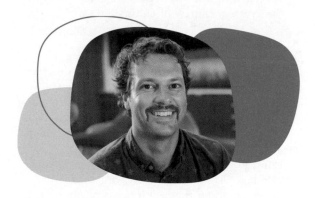

Simon's story

 View Simon's story or read the transcript.

Simon is a father of three children. He talks about his experience of becoming a father and how the midwives actively engaged him. He also gives some advice on ways that midwives can actively engage fathers.

Reflection

1. Reflect on what the midwives did to encourage Simon to be engaged, particularly around the birth of his first child and the early parenting period.

2. What are some of the issues and challenges for fathers identified by Simon?

Inquiry

1. Fathers who share the care of their children or become the primary carer often identify that there are not the same social support networks available to them as for mothers. Identify some relevant community and professional resources and support services for fathers in your area.

2. Access The Fatherhood Institute at www.fatherhoodinstitute.org and read the discussion on fathers and maternity care. What are some important practice points for midwives when considering new fathers?

3. Fathers play an important role in breastfeeding and support. Search for the literature on fathers and breastfeeding (see resource list below) and discuss the ways in which the father's unique circumstances could have an impact on involvement and support.

Action

Since fathers are important influencers of mothers' health choices and experiences before, during and after the birth, it benefits the whole family when maternity professionals make fathers feel welcomed and involved and prepare them for their role at the birth and afterwards.

1. Discuss with your colleagues strategies that midwives can use to engage men in the parenting role, particularly men from marginalised backgrounds.

2. Visit the Men and Parenting Pathways website at mappresearch.org and explore the resources. Write a list of five things that may impact the father's ability to provide support during the pregnancy, birth and postnatal period and consider how you might broach these topics at an antenatal visit.

A FINAL WORD

There are many benefits of positively engaging fathers during pregnancy, birth and postpartum periods such as an improvement in breastfeeding rates and maternal mental health. Midwives should take every opportunity to provide relevant and up-to-date information, guidance and support to enable fathers to be actively involved.

Resources

Men and Parenting Pathways: http://mappresearch.org/
The Fatherhood Institute: http://www.fatherhoodinstitute.org/

CHAPTER 12

Multiple pregnancy

INTRODUCTION

Multiple births have increased in developed countries over the past 30 years, mainly due to the prevalence of assisted reproductive techniques and older women having babies. The number of multiple births in Australia has remained stable at around 2–3% of all births (from 3.1% (9442) of births in 2010 to 2.9% (8469) of births in 2020) (Australian Institute of Health and Welfare, 2022). In 2020 almost all multiple births (98%) were twins, and 2% were other multiples (triplets, quadruplets or higher) (Australian Institute of Health and Welfare, 2022).

There are two types of twin pregnancies: dizygotic and monozygotic.
*   Dizygotic twins have separate sacs, placentae and membranes (chorion and amnion), and are developed from two different spermatozoa and ova. They can be of the same or different sex, and are similar in likeness to siblings.
*   Monozygotic babies develop from the same fertilised ovum. This ovum splits into two identical halves; hence, the twins are of the same sex and look similar to each other. They share the same placenta and chorion membrane, and mostly have a separate amnion (Macdonald et al., 2017).

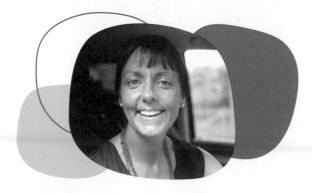

Cassandre's story

 View Cassandre's story or read the transcript.

Cassandre has had two sets of twins. She describes her decision making regarding her mode of birth and the factors that influenced her decision. She also describes the care she received at the time of the birth, in particular the emotional support that helped her (sections 1, 2 and 4). In sections 3 and 5 of Cassandre's story, she talks about communication, family support and being labelled as 'high risk'.

Reflection

Women with a multiple pregnancy have an increased risk of complications, which can affect the health of the mother and her babies.
1. Listen to Cassandre's experience of care during her pregnancy and birth. What was it that she felt was missing in her care?
2. For her first set of twins, Cassandre was given advice (which was not evidence based) that

steered her towards thinking a caesarean section would be more appropriate for her. Cassandre states that she was told she 'probably would have to have a C-section' for the birth of her second twin. What could have been improved in the choices she was given regarding the mode of birth?

3. Understand how Cassandre felt when being labelled as 'high risk' and listen to her personal strategies on how to deal with that in her second twin pregnancy.

4. Cassandre discusses her postnatal care after her first set of twins. Reflect on the flexibility of the hospital staff to relax hospital policies so as to facilitate family support. What happens in your clinical workplace when a new mother with twins is admitted to the postnatal ward? In what other postnatal situations should women be allowed to have extended visiting hours (e.g. partner staying overnight) so that she can have extra family support?

5. How would you feel if you were told you were expecting twins and you already had twin toddlers at home? List the feelings you would expect to have and the support you would like from your midwife.

6. Think about the differences in the care Cassandre received in her pregnancies. What main qualities did the midwives have that Cassandre appreciated?

7. Imagine you are told that you are a high-risk woman during your antenatal clinic visits. Document how would this make you feel? What strategies did Cassandre employ to deal with this label?

Inquiry

1. Find the Cochrane Library online and search for a trial on planned caesarean section for a twin pregnancy. Find out how many women have emergency caesarean sections for their second twins (note this in relation to the advice Cassandre received about the mode of birth).

2. Health professionals and pregnant women understand risk differently. Look up and read the following article: 'The tensions of uncertainty: Midwives managing risk in and of their practice' (Skinner & Maude, 2016).

3. Look on the Australian Multiple Birth Association website: http://www.amba.org.au. Find the page 'Looking for support—expecting multiples' and reflect on how this association can be of great help to parents expecting twins.

4. With her first set of twins, Cassandre was unable to walk to the special care nursery to see her babies, and she states that it was difficult to find a midwife to bring one of her babies to her for feeds. Look up the definition of 'woman-centred care' in the Code of Conduct for Midwives (NMBA, 2018). Were midwives caring for Cassandre in this way?

5. Explore the 'high-risk' element to multiple pregnancies. What are the main complications that can accompany a multiple pregnancy and birth? Have a look at the website 'Health Direct' for information about complications in pregnancy (https://www.healthdirect.gov.au/pregnancy-complications).

6. Ensure you have balanced, current, evidence-based information regarding mode of birth for women with multiple pregnancies. Mode of birth needs to be taken into account, including the gestation, lie, presentation and estimated size of the babies, together with any other fetal or maternal health risks and, most importantly, the woman's preference.

7. Role-play with a peer a discussion between a woman with a twin pregnancy and a midwife regarding the pros and cons of different modes of birth, and the midwifery support she would need.

8. Find a specific resource on the Australian Breastfeeding Association website (https://www.breastfeeding.asn.au) that would help support women who are breastfeeding multiples.

9. Breastfeeding policy promotes baby-led feeding. Discuss with a peer why Cassandre did not completely follow this recommendation.

A FINAL WORD

There are higher risks involved when the mother has a multiple pregnancy. These are an increased risk of anaemia, hypertensive disorders, miscarriage, caesarean section, haemorrhage and breastfeeding challenges. Because of these factors, midwifery and obstetric support is vital for women having multiples. However, women with multiple pregnancies, like Cassandre, will also need individually tailored, woman-centred midwifery care, with current evidence-based information regarding the most appropriate mode of birth. Quality postnatal care and family involvement are also very important in relation to establishing breastfeeding and encouraging essential support networks.

CHAPTER 13

Perinatal mental health

INTRODUCTION

Mental health disorders in the perinatal period are common and occur during pregnancy and the first year after birth; perinatal depression affects mother–infant interactions, making it a public health concern (Bernard et al., 2018). Perinatal mental health disorders have also been associated with increased rates of preterm birth. Recent research suggests that around 15–22% of women experience depression during pregnancy and/or following the birth of their baby (Bryson et al., 2021; Dennis et al., 2017); furthermore, one to two women per 1000 women giving birth will experience postnatal psychosis (VanderKruik et al., 2017). It has also been proposed that one in five women report anxiety symptoms during pregnancy, and between 4% and 20% of women experience symptoms of an anxiety disorder after giving birth (Leach & Fairweather-Schmidt, 2017). It has also been estimated that between 3% and 4.2% of women will experience both anxiety and depression (Falah-Hassani et al., 2017) and, therefore, it is essential that midwives prioritise screening for mental health concerns and caring for these women in pregnancy.

If a woman experiences depression during the perinatal period, it can have severe consequences, not only for the woman experiencing it but also for her children and family (Marmorstein et al., 2004). Perinatal mental health disorders have been associated with increased rates of preterm birth (Dayan et al., 2006), increased infant crying (Wormser et al., 2006) and a negative impact on the infant's cognitive, emotional and behavioural development (Milgrom et al., 2004).

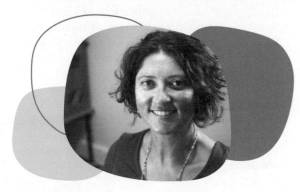

Kathryn's story

 View Kathryn's story or read the transcript.

Kathryn is a clinical nurse consultant in perinatal and infant mental health. Her story describes perinatal mental health disorders, signs and symptoms, and which women are more likely to experience perinatal mental health concerns. Kathy also describes the recommended midwifery care (sections 1 and 2) and the management (sections 3 and 4).

Reflection

1. Postpartum depression can be classified in five domains of risk factors: psychiatric, obstetric, biological and hormonal, social and lifestyle. Low education and income are associated with a higher risk of postpartum depression. What other pregnancy complications are women with these backgrounds predisposed to?

33

2. Watch this video from PANDA that presents real-life stories of parents who have experienced postnatal depression (PND) and anxiety: 'Behind the Mask: The hidden struggle of parenthood' on https://www.youtube.com/watch?v=FjqOqJLkyFs.

3. Kathryn talks about the shame women feel when they have mental health disorders. How might this be related to the pressure felt by parents to be perfect mothers and fathers? Read this article on the subject from the American Sociological Association: http://www.asanet.org/press/super_parent_cultural_pressures.cfm.

4. Exercise (even a single bout of activity) has been found to be helpful to increase mood and self-esteem in people experiencing poor mental health. How do you talk to women about exercise during pregnancy?

Inquiry

1. Women may present with a number of different perinatal mental health disorders. List the common disorders and write a few sentences about each one stating the presenting symptoms.

2. Name the common anti-anxiety or antidepressant medications used for pregnant or breastfeeding women? What medications do pregnant or breastfeeding women take for bipolar disorder or schizophrenia? Look at the Australian Therapeutic Goods Administration (TGA) website for information about prescribing medicines in pregnancy: https://www.tga.gov.au/australian-categorisation-system-prescribing-medicines-pregnancy.

3. Major perinatal mental health disorders can involve suicidal thoughts and suicide attempts. Suicide is a leading contributor to maternal mortality worldwide and is strongly associated with violence and abuse (Rahman et al., 2013). Look at the recent Australian maternal mortality report: https://www.aihw.gov.au/reports/mothers-babies/maternal-deaths-australia. How many maternal deaths in the period 2010 to 2021 were due to suicide?

4. Despite many years of research aimed at identifying the causes of PND (sometimes known as postpartum depression or PPD), PND remains common and no definitive causes have been found. Kathryn discusses the 'protective factors' women have: what are these?

5. Antidepressants are often warranted but treatment needs to be holistic, including counselling, complementary therapies and social support, among other treatments. Antidepressants alone may not fully address the issues. Review the COPE *Mental Health Care in the Perinatal Period: Australian Clinical Practice Guideline* (COPE, 2017, pp. 50–51) to see what the recommendations for complementary therapies such as omega-3 fatty acids, St John's Wort, Ginkgo biloba and acupuncture are.

Action

1. Postpartum psychosis is a relatively rare event with a range of estimated incidence of 1.1 to 4.0 cases per 1000 deliveries. Kathryn discusses some symptoms women have when this condition presents. Look at this website: https://www.cope.org.au/new-parents/postnatal-mental-health-conditions/postpatum-psychosis/ and read the information on postpartum psychosis. What are the early signs of postpartum psychosis? Look at the Edinburgh Postnatal Depression Scale (EPDS): https://www.cope.org.au/health-professionals/health-professionals-3/calculating-score-epds/. Become familiar with the questions and how the scoring works. In particular, if women score 1, 2 or 3 on question 10, you need to enquire further about her safety and, if concerned, contact senior staff for help. At what other times in the perinatal period are women screened with the EPDS?

2. Go to the Beyondblue website and click on this link about perinatal anxiety: https://healthyfamilies.beyondblue.org.au/pregnancy-and-new-parents/maternal-mental-health-and-wellbeing/anxiety. Then click on this link about resources for women: https://healthyfamilies.beyondblue.org.au/seeking-support/professional-support/support-from-health-professionals. Kathryn discusses how midwives can also help when women demonstrate mild anxiety (e.g. about the birth process). Have a discussion with your peers about how they talk with women about birth.

3. Make sure you know what resources are available to women and families so that you can inform the women in your care. Here is a link to resources: https://healthyfamilies.beyondblue.org.au/seeking-support/professional-support/helpful-contacts-and-websites.

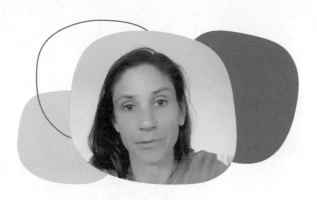

Amy's story

 View Amy's story or read the transcript.

Amy is a 39-year-old woman who is married and the mother of four children. In this story, Amy shares her pregnancy, birth and postnatal experience with her third baby, Freya. Amy shares her experience of having anxiety and depression postnatally and gives insight into ways that midwives can better support women.

Reflection

1. Amy describes the care provided by her midwives on the home birth program. Reflect on how this care could have been improved to make Amy feel less anxious about the birth and postnatal period.

2. Amy describes signs and symptoms of anxiety and postnatal depression. Reflect on how you might respond to Amy if she disclosed this information to you in a midwifery appointment.

3. Reflect on how Amy's mental health impacted on the relationship she had with her husband, other children and baby Freya.

Inquiry

1. Familiarise yourself with guideline 6.71 'Perinatal mental health concerns' from the Australian College of Midwives' *National Midwifery Guidelines for Consultation and Referral* (2021).

2. Visit the 'MumMoodBooster' website: https://mummoodbooster.com/public/ and become familiar with this Australian evidence-based treatment program for postnatal depression.

3. Find out what support services are available for women and healthcare professionals in your local area: https://www.cope.org.au/

Action

1. View the Centre of Perinatal Excellence (COPE) #thetruth video series and watch the early parenthood video at https://www.cope.org.au/thetruth/.

2. Amy describes the support, care and medications that helped to support her through the postnatal period. Write a list of these and add any other resources available to women in your local area; for example, mother-and-baby units or other private facilities.

3. List the supportive midwifery actions and helpful advice that Amy discusses and consider how you could incorporate these into your midwifery care.

A FINAL WORD

Perinatal mental health disorders are common, debilitating and come at a time when parents expect joy and delight at the birth of their baby. In fact, women are more likely to be affected by depression and anxiety during pregnancy and childbirth than at any other time in their lives. Midwives play an important role in screening and referring women who are at risk. Working in continuity of care models and having a relationship with women during pregnancy, birth and the postnatal period can help midwives to identify issues early and provide timely assessment and referral.

CHAPTER 14
Complex pregnancies

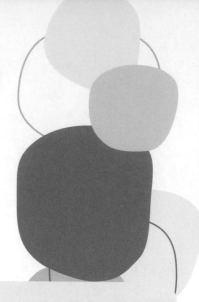

INTRODUCTION

This chapter introduces you to a woman who develops complexities in pregnancy. Preeclampsia is a complication of pregnancy associated with new-onset high blood pressure complicating around 3–5% of all pregnancies (Chappell et al., 2021; 'Gestational Hypertension and Preeclampsia', 2020). Guidelines have been developed for consistency in the definition and midwifery/medical management of hypertensive disorders in pregnancy (Lowe, 2014). Women with preeclampsia often have their labour induced or undergo a caesarean section before their due date, meaning their babies are born early (Lowe, 2014). Premature birth is the leading cause of neonatal death and disability (World Health Organization, 2018). Advancement in neonatal intensive care has improved outcomes for babies in countries that have these services (WHO, 2018). The experience for women and their families of having a baby in the neonatal intensive care can be very difficult, as Trish describes.

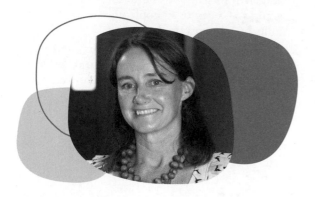

Trish's story

 View Trish's story or read the transcript.

Trish talks about being pregnant with twins. She booked with an obstetrician to provide care and to be available for the birth as she understands there are complexities with a twin pregnancy. Trish was upset when her hopes of having a natural labour were shattered early in the pregnancy when the obstetrician explained that he would like her to have an epidural. Trish accepted the obstetrician's position and understood that there may be a need for an emergency caesarean between babies.

The pregnancy progressed well until around 30 weeks, when Trish was diagnosed with rapid-onset hypertension and preeclampsia and admitted to hospital. With worsening preeclampsia, Trish faced the prospect of having her twins prematurely.

Reflection

1. In her opening discussion, Trish talks about how her pregnancy was progressing quite normally and that she was still working.

Consider the impact on women's lives when the pregnancy becomes unexpectedly complicated by a disease such as preeclampsia. Think about how a woman's life can be put into disarray with a diagnosis of preeclampsia and admission to hospital.

2. The paediatrician prepared Trish for how her babies would look when born early and the care they would receive, along with giving her a tour of the neonatal intensive care unit. What midwifery actions could assist women to prepare for a premature birth?

3. An emergency caesarean for a life-threatening condition can be a frightening experience for a mother. Think of ways you can support women who are given this news.

4. Trish was able to have skin-to-skin contact with her babies in the operating theatre. Think about how this may have helped Trish to initiate and maintain breastfeeding.

5. What helped Trish in the first few days after the birth when she went to visit the babies in the nursery?

Inquiry

1. Trish's discussion of her hospitalisation illustrates how she was trying to second-guess the decision around her health and the likely preterm birth of her babies. Read the study titled 'Experiences of women with hypertensive disorders of pregnancy: A scoping review' (Sakurai et al., 2022). Think about what information would have improved Trish's experience of being hospitalised.

2. How did the midwife support Trish when the decision was made to have the babies?

3. How did Trish describe all the people at the birth?

4. From Trish's perspective, what was important to her at the birth?

5. Read the article 'Parental experiences of family-centred care from admission to discharge in the neonatal intensive care unit' (Serlachius

et al., 2018). How did Trish describe the nurses in the neonatal intensive care unit? What qualities did she find helpful?

6. What was helpful to Trish in establishing breastfeeding?

7. What supports did Trish have when she went home?

8. What did Trish value the most when she came home with the boys?

Action

A woman is admitted with preeclampsia from home. She is accompanied by her husband.

1. Write down how you would approach the woman and her husband and write a brief list of topics you would discuss with them.

2. Consider providing the woman with written information. Where would you access online/written information to help the woman understand the diagnosis of preeclampsia, the need for hospitalisation and the likely outcomes of pregnancy?

3. Write a list of the professionals you (as the midwife) need to consult and refer with in order to provide comprehensive care for the woman and her family.

4. Revise your emergency response to an eclamptic seizure.

5. How would you prepare a woman and her partner for the unexpected yet planned preterm birth of their baby/babies?

6. Write a synopsis of the likely outcomes for babies born in Australia, at 24, 26, 28, 30 and 32 weeks' gestation.

7. Discuss the implications for establishing breastfeeding.

8. What resources would you source to guide your practice in relation to consultation and referral?

Text links

Chapter 37, 'Challenges in Pregnancy', *Midwifery: Preparation for Practice* (5th ed.) (Pairman et al., 2022).

FINAL WORD

The development of preeclampsia in pregnancy can be a life-threatening and frightening experience for women as they face hospitalisation and an induced early birth. Trish describes how the midwifery, obstetric and paediatric staff supported her in hospital. Trish particularly felt prepared for how the babies would look and the care they would receive in the neonatal nursery as she was counselled by the paediatrician and had a tour of the neonatal intensive care unit. Trish also describes being well supported by her midwifery friend and husband. It is important to remember, even in life-threatening emergencies, the importance of the woman's support people. Trish describes the nurses caring for her premature babies as kind and involving her, as a mother, in the care of her twin babies. Trish really appreciated having skin-to-skin contact with the babies whenever possible and attributes her success in establishing breastfeeding to this action. The other support was home visiting by a midwife once the boys were home. Together, the midwifery and family support helped Trish gain confidence in early mothering and in establishing and maintaining breastfeeding.

CHAPTER 15
Grief and loss

INTRODUCTION

The following chapter will discuss grief and loss in maternity care, including miscarriage, stillbirth and moving forward into the future. The first section focuses on one couple's story about the birth of their stillborn baby, and another woman's experience of having further children following the stillbirth of her twin daughters. Many women are not given enough information from their maternity care provider about recognising normal fetal movements and, more importantly, to contact their maternity care provider when they perceive decreased fetal movements (Rumbold et al., 2020). Consequently, several guidelines have been written for maternity care providers that help them give women information about decreased fetal movements and the need for further investigations (Rumbold et al., 2020). Decreased fetal movements are recognised as a warning sign that placental function may be impaired (Rumbold et al., 2020). It is for this reason that women should be advised to contact their midwife or other care provider if they experience any changes in the fetal movements.

The last section of this chapter provides an overview of early pregnancy loss from the perspective of a midwife, Nikki, who works in an Early Pregnancy Assessment Service (EPAS). The EPAS unit offers assessment of early pregnancy complications and management of early pregnancy loss (Lee, 2022). Early pregnancy complications are very distressing experiences for women and include bleeding in pregnancy, ectopic pregnancy and miscarriage. Approximately 20–40% of women will experience bleeding in early pregnancy; however, only around 20% of women will experience miscarriage (Pairman et al., 2022). Miscarriage and early pregnancy loss are very distressing for women and their families, resulting in feelings of grief and loss.

Miscarriage is defined as pregnancy loss before 20 weeks' gestation, where the fetus weighs less than 400 grams (Pairman et al., 2022). The arbitrary definition is designed to assist parents with the understanding of their pregnancy loss, and clinicians with deciding on the best course of treatment at the time; however, it does not consider the associated grief and loss parents experience. Some miscarriages result in infection and can be life-threatening. This condition is called septic miscarriage. Early pregnancy bleeding can also be caused by an ectopic pregnancy, defined as the implantation of a fertilised ovum in a site other than the endometrium of the uterus (Pairman et al., 2022). An ectopic pregnancy occurs in about 1–2% of all pregnancies, causes a lot of pain and, if ruptured, can be life threatening for the woman (Pairman et al., 2022). Care must include ensuring women know how to contact their midwife as soon as any bleeding is noted in pregnancy so they can be referred to an EPAS unit.

The terms *abortion* and *miscarriage* are often used interchangeably, and this can cause confusion to women who think of an abortion as purposefully ending a pregnancy before 20 weeks rather than as a spontaneous loss. This can be a confronting and medicalised term to use with women who are grieving the loss of their baby. A systematic review demonstrated a gap in psychological support for women following miscarriage with the risk of the woman experiencing anxiety and depression (Ho et al.,

2022). The authors also found that care provided in ambulatory care clinics had a more streamlined approach to diagnosis and treatment options in the presence of supportive staff, similar to the EPAS clinic that Nikki describes later in this chapter.

A ten-year retrospective study conducted in Canada evaluated the sustained value of an Early Pregnancy Assessment Clinic in the management of early pregnancy complications and the effect on the incidence emergency room (ER) visits (Pinnaduwage et al., 2018). The study included over 10,000 women and found the early pregnancy assessment clinic is a vital service for managing early pregnancy complications for women. However, the clinic has not yet had a sustained impact on visits to the emergency rooms for miscarriage, ectopic pregnancy and haemorrhage, and the authors recommend a clinic available to women every day.

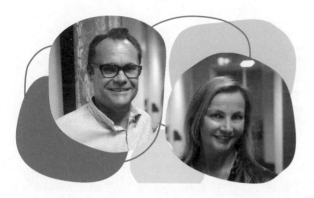

Ali and David's story

 View Ali and David's story or read the transcript.

Ali and David describe their excitement about becoming parents for the first time. There had been no complications in their pregnancy and they expected to give birth in a midwife-led birth centre. Ali states that there was a change in the baby's movements at around 32 weeks. When Ali contacted her midwife, she was given the correct advice to come to the birth centre for further investigation.

Reflection

1. Think about how you might respond to a woman who has a perception that something has changed with the baby, in particular the woman's perceptions of fetal movements.

2. Think about what phrases or comments are helpful to the parents of a newly discovered fetal death in utero.

3. Ali and David were advised to go home and then come back the following day to have the labour induced. Ali states that she did not think she could give birth to a 'dead' child, and it was the words of her care providers that gave her the confidence to give birth just as she had planned. Think about how you might discuss birth choices with a woman who has experienced a fetal death in utero. Reflect on Ali's thoughts regarding a caesarean.

4. David describes the staff as subdued around the time of birth and says that the experience of stillbirth is very quiet as there is no baby crying. David states that in this situation he remembers all the things people say—both the good things and the not-so-good things. Reflect on what was helpful for Ali and David to hear regarding their daughter, Harper.

5. Ali and David discuss the birth surroundings. Think about what was helpful about their birth environment.

Inquiry

1. Explore the Stillbirth Centre of Research Excellence found here: https://stillbirthcre.org.au/.

2. Its purpose is to develop a deeper understanding of the impact of stillbirth on families, midwives and other care providers and develop skills in understanding some of the causes of and what can be done to try to prevent stillbirth.

3. Develop strategies to assist your midwifery practice by enhancing the knowledge of pregnant women about reporting their baby's movements.

4. David discusses wanting to stay in hospital so that the medical people can 'fix this'. He says that this is a masculine or male way of looking at things. Read the article 'New understandings of fathers' experiences of grief and loss

following stillbirth and neonatal death: A scoping review' (Jones et al., 2019) and think about how David and other fathers grieve following the death of their baby.

5. What did the midwives do when Ali and David were in labour with Harper that made them feel so special and important?

6. Discuss how you may make women feel that they are able to give birth naturally, even in the case of fetal demise. What can you do for the father to make them feel that they still have a fathering role in the birth of their deceased child?

7. Write a list of some actions/words that a midwife can use when providing care to the baby post-birth.

8. Discuss who you will refer the parents to during or immediately after the birth process.

Action

You are providing care to a couple who have experienced fetal demise.

1. Discuss how you will respond to these parents initially.

2. Refer to the Australian College of Midwives' *National Midwifery Guidelines for Consultation and Referral* (Australian College of Midwives, 2021) in relation to stillbirth. What referral process do you have in your place of midwifery practice when providing care to a family that experiences stillbirth?

3. How will you discuss/plan the birth for these parents? What do you need to consider in your discussion of the birth plan?

4. Immediately following birth, what midwifery care would assist the parents at this intimate and sad time?

5. In the postnatal period, how are you going to provide midwifery care to the mother?

6. Who else would you offer to provide care to the woman?

7. What kind of memories/keepsakes will you provide to the parents?

8. How will you look after your own feelings when you experience such a sad event in your midwifery practice?

Text links

Chapter 43, 'Grief and loss during childbearing – the crying times', *Midwifery: Preparation for Practice*, 5th ed. (Pairman et al., 2022).

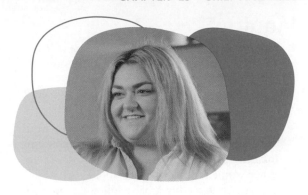

Ashleigh's story

 View Ashleigh's story or read the transcript.

Ashleigh shares her experience of giving birth to baby Florence following the previous loss of stillborn twin daughters. Ashleigh shares her conflicting feelings of fear and excitement that she experienced throughout her pregnancy with Florence, and the positive support she received from her obstetrician, the midwives, as well as her husband and close family and friends. Ashleigh provides a positive message of hope to other women who go on to have a baby following previous infant loss.

Reflection

1. Ashleigh expressed feeling both fear and excitement when she found out she was pregnant with Florence. Reflect on the rollercoaster of emotions that women may feel throughout the different stages of the childbearing journey when they find out they are pregnant following previous infant loss.

2. Think about how you might provide sensitive, woman-centred care in your midwifery practice for women who have fallen pregnant after a previous infant loss. How can you help these women feel supported? What language might you use?

3. Ashleigh highlighted the importance of seeking professional help through therapy as a way to resolve the guilt she felt and process her emotions about both her previous stillbirth and her subsequent pregnancy with Florence. In what other ways could professional therapy or counselling be beneficial for women having a baby following previous infant loss?

Inquiry

1. Which of the NMBA *Midwife Standards for Practice* (2018) best relate to the provision of sensitive, individualised and supportive midwifery care for women who are pregnant following previous infant loss?

2. Would giving birth to a subsequent baby heal the grief experienced from the previous infant loss? Why or why not? See if you can look up other women's stories online about their experience of having a baby following previous stillbirth or infant loss.

3. Does a previous stillbirth increase risks for the mother or baby in a subsequent pregnancy? Research this issue and list any potential risks you find.

Action

1. Consider the importance of support for women who have a subsequent pregnancy following previous infant loss. Search online to find organisations or local support groups that provide resources and support to women in this situation. What can you find?

2. Write a list of the ways midwives, obstetricians and the health service can adequately support women (and their partners) to feel reassured and supported during a subsequent pregnancy after infant loss.

3. Partners/fathers are poorly represented in the literature in relation to their own feelings of grief following infant loss. Read the following article that examines parents' concerns (mothers and fathers) about future pregnancy after stillbirth (Meaney et al., 2017): https://onlinelibrary.wiley.com/doi/full/10.1111/hex.12480.

4. Babies born after a previous infant loss are often referred to as 'rainbow' babies. Some women, however, may prefer not to use this term. As midwives we need to ensure our language is respectful of the woman's preferences, particularly in sensitive situations. Read the following article (Hanson, 2022) where mother Teresa Mendoza explains the reasons why she prefers not to use the term rainbow baby: https://www.today.com/parents/rainbow-baby-why-some-parents-dislike-term-t233195.

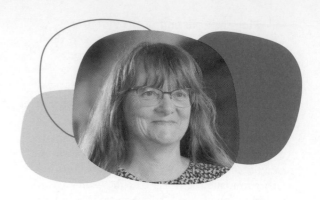

Nikki's story

 View Nikki's story or read the transcript.

Nikki discusses how the emergency department can't always provide the midwifery support that is offered through the early pregnancy assessment unit. The EPAS unit can arrange blood tests and ultrasounds while women are in the non-acute stage while supported by the midwife. The support continues after the event with Nikki providing her name and telephone contact to the women together with written material. Nikki invites the women to contact her if they have any questions, concerns or worries. This exemplary service provided by a skilled, knowledgeable midwife is very important for women and their families at such a devastating time of grief and loss.

Reflection

1. Think about how Nikki describes being a support to women during their experience of early pregnancy complications. How do you think this support differs from the support provided in an emergency room?

2. Reflect on Nikki's recommendations for self-care and how important self-care is for midwives working in an EPAS unit.

3. Think about how women and their families are feeling when they experience a miscarriage and what supports would be useful to them.

Inquiry

1. Read the section titled 'Bleeding in Early Pregnancy' in Chapter 37 of the text *Midwifery:*

Preparation for Practice, 5th ed (Pairman et al., 2022) and define the following:

a. Threatened miscarriage

b. Inevitable (imminent) miscarriage

c. Complete miscarriage

d. Incomplete miscarriage

e. Silent or delayed miscarriage (missed abortion, blood mole, carneous mole or stony/fleshy mole)

f. Record the sites where ectopic pregnancies can be found and list the signs and symptoms

2. Think about the times as a midwifery student when you may require extra support and where you may be able to access that support. Make a list for ease of reference.

Action

1. Write a list of the self-care practices that you engage in when you are feeling sad or overwhelmed from a midwifery professional experience placement experience or even a personal experience of loss and grief.

2. Think of and write a list of three *new* places to find support that you have never accessed before.

3. Look for the EPAS clinic in the maternity service where you are undertaking midwifery professional experience practice. If you do not have an EPAS unit, search the internet to find out where the closest unit is from your placement site.

4. Discuss the use of the Australian College of Midwives' National Midwifery Guidelines for Consultation and Referral (2021) when midwives are providing care for women in early pregnancy. What category does bleeding in early pregnancy come under? A, B or C?

5. When taking a history from a woman at the first visit, discuss how you would respond to a woman who has experienced a previous miscarriage.

6. Using the Nursing and Midwifery Board of Australia's *Midwife Standards for Practice* (2018), write a brief synopsis on how Nikki's role in the EPAS unit meets the standards for practice.

Text link

Chapter 37, 'Challenges in pregnancy' in *Midwifery: Preparation for Practice*, 5th ed. (Pairman et al., 2022).

A FINAL WORD

This chapter has explored the profound impact of pregnancy loss from the perspectives of women, partners and midwives. Miscarriage and stillbirth continue to remain topics often not spoken about, adding a hidden layer of emotional grief following the loss of a baby. Future pregnancies following loss can be filled with varying emotions, from excitement and happiness to fear and anxiety. The stories in this chapter have given us insight into what women and their partners appreciated from the midwives and doctors who provided care to them through this very challenging time in their lives. Remembering to acknowledge the baby as a person, irrespective of the gestation in which it was lost, is important for those who have experienced miscarriage or stillbirth. It is also important to remember that not every woman who experiences stillbirth will have positive memories of the birth experience and in your midwifery care you need to explore the woman's experience sensitively without assumption.

CHAPTER 16

Assisted reproductive technologies

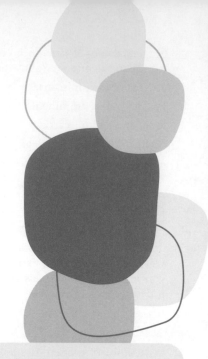

INTRODUCTION

In Australia in 2011, over 88,900 women undertook some form of ART to achieve a pregnancy, resulting in 17–28% women having live births (Newman, 2021). The prevalence of women seeking fertility treatments is increasing, as are the number of clinics and types of ART available. Midwives care for many women who have undertaken some form of fertility treatment, and it is important to understand what this means from the perspective of the midwife and the woman.

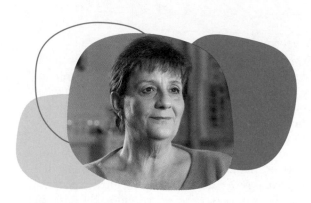

midwifery care of couples undergoing ART. Lastly, she describes a typical day in her role as clinical midwifery specialist.

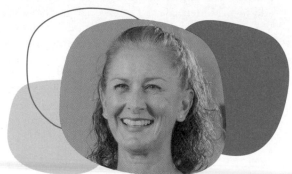

Sandra's story

 View Sandra's story or read the transcript.

Sections 1 to 3 of Sandra's story describe the reasons for and some types of ART available, what women experience and the financial implications of having this treatment. In section 4, Sandra describes the

Robyn's story

 View Robyn's story or read the transcript.

Robyn describes her journey to becoming a single mother of twins using ART.

Reflection

1. Pre-implantation genetic diagnoses are questionable to some people, and there are ethical implications. Why would this be?

2. Many older women have children with the help of ART. What complications can occur in these circumstances?

3. Reflect on the emotional experience and financial implications for women undergoing ART.

4. Sandra mentions that if the woman discloses that she has had fertility treatment during a booking visit, it is important to ascertain how many cycles she has had. Why does she say this is important?

5. Robyn describes having very good care throughout her pregnancy and birth except for one incident with a health professional. What was this incident and how do you think it could have been improved?

Inquiry

1. Sandra mentions that age, weight and male sperm production are three reasons why women may have difficulty achieving a pregnancy. What are the other causes of infertility?

2. Write a dot-point list of all the different types of ART. Summarise the method in a couple of sentences underneath each point.

3. Are there different rules across the States and Territories of Australia relating to access to ART?

4. What is the recommended period of time for women to wait before obtaining help with fertility? Why is this recommendation different for women over 35 years of age?

5. Investigate the medicines that are used to treat infertility in women. These all have side effects. Through your institutional library, look up clomiphene citrate in MIMS Online and list the side effects of this medication.

Action

1. Find a service near you that provides fertility treatment. How much does each treatment cost? What Medicare rebates are available?

2. There are some natural fertility-boosting methods available to couples. Find out what these are and whether there is existing evidence to support their use.

3. Go to https://npesu.unsw.cdu.au/sites/default/files/npesu/surveillances/Assisted%20 Reproductive%20Technology%20in%20 Australia%20and%20New%20Zealand%20 2019.pdf (Newman et al., 2021) and read the summary of this annual report that outlines the prevalence and success of ART in Australia and New Zealand.

4. Go to https://www.cochrane.org/CD012692/MENSTR_interventions-unexplained-infertility-systematic-review-and-meta-analysis (Wang et al., 2019). This describes the evidence surrounding different treatments for infertility.

A FINAL WORD

Increasingly, couples and singles are using ART to help achieve pregnancy and, ultimately, a live birth. There are many different infertility treatments available. They are costly and emotionally and physically draining. Sandra gives a good account of the challenges and complexities midwives face working with these couples. Robyn gives an excellent account of what the process is like as a single woman wanting to become a mother. When caring for women who have undergone fertility treatment, midwives need to acknowledge these difficulties and tailor their care accordingly.

CHAPTER 17

Vaginal birth after caesarean section

INTRODUCTION

This chapter tells the story of a woman choosing to have a vaginal birth following a caesarean section for her first birth. There are rising caesarean section rates for women in Australia and the cause for this rise is difficult to determine (AIWH, 2022). It has been proposed that caesarean section rates have been influenced by clinical decision making, medico-legal concerns or maternal request (ACSQHC, 2021; AIHW, 2022). It is evident that women who are privately insured have a higher chance of having a caesarean section (Dahlen et al., 2014; Miller et al., 2022). With the rising rates of caesarean section, decision making regarding the next mode of birth becomes important. Having a vaginal birth after a previous caesarean is generally considered safe for many women; however, there are numerous considerations that must be taken into account when making the decision as to mode of next birth. When determining which option may be safer and less harmful for the mother and/or baby, these considerations should be discussed with the woman by her primary caregiver in consideration of any risk factors that may be present (Devarajan et al., 2018). It is acknowledged that the decisions about mode of birth following a previous caesarean section are complex for women. Women will balance both risk versus chance in the context of their own individual circumstances. To help women through this decision-making process, supportive care providers, especially midwives, are important (Davis et al., 2020). Evidence has shown that vaginal birth after caesarean section is the more cost-effective option for the health system compared with elective repeat caesarean sections (Fobelets et al., 2018). Guidelines have been developed to help maternity service providers discuss the next mode of birth with women who have had a previous caesarean section (The Royal Hospital for Women, 2022).

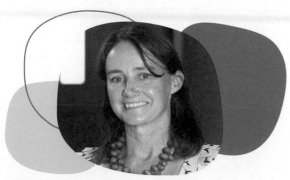

Trish's story

 View Trish's story or read the transcript.

Trish tells the story of accessing a private obstetrician for her pregnancy and birth care with her next baby, following a caesarean section. She describes the difficulty she had convincing the private obstetrician to support her to have a vaginal birth after caesarean. Trish researched the safety and accessed information through her friend, a midwife. It was this action that meant she could try for a vaginal birth after caesarean. In addition, Trish received continuity of midwifery care from a midwifery student for this pregnancy and birth. Trish felt the obstetrician provided her with a lot of information and discussed options with her; however, there was always a need to negotiate in order to have the birth Trish planned.

Reflection

1. Think about the language midwives and obstetricians use with women when discussing vaginal birth after caesarean section. Trish describes the doctor as not letting her go over term and the doctor saying 'you're allowed to do this, but then at that point, you're not allowed to'. How do you think the language used impacts women's decision making around their mode of birth?

2. Trish says the doctor would not let her go over her due date and also refused to do a stretch and sweep on her due date. Think about the evidence for having a stretch and sweep at term to prevent induction of labour (Finucane et al., 2020) or, in this case, a repeat caesarean section for Trish.

3. Trish discusses how the doctor told her, when she was in labour, she had until midday and that she felt she had no say in the decision-making process. How could the doctor or midwife discuss how much time in labour would be appropriate for a woman having a vaginal birth after caesarean?

4. Trish describes the difference in recovery from a caesarean to a vaginal birth, in particular the pain she experienced. Think about discussing pain following a surgical birth with the pain women experience in labour, and how the women are able to care for their babies following both modes of birth.

Inquiry

1. What is the role of a midwife when a woman approaches you requesting a vaginal birth after caesarean section?

2. What do the Australian College of Midwives' *National Midwifery Guidelines for Consultation and Referral* (2021) state in regard to collaboration and referral for women choosing a vaginal birth following caesarean?

3. How can you ensure that the information you provide for the woman is evidence-based and free from bias, with regard to safety for the mother and baby? What factors need to be considered when discussing benefits versus risk with the woman?

4. What is the benefit of having support in labour from a known caregiver (midwifery continuity of care) on the rate of caesarean sections (Betrán et al., 2018)?

Action

1. Write a synopsis on how to support women to avoid the primary (first) caesarean section.

2. Write a list of discussion points you need to have with a woman about her first caesarean section that will enable you to provide unbiased information for deciding on her next mode of birth.

3. Develop a decision-making tool (such as a pamphlet, a short YouTube video or a list of the issues you would discuss with a woman in a one-on-one counselling session) on the pros and cons of a repeat caesarean section.

4. Write a role play using language that enables women to make an informed decision when deciding on either a repeat caesarean section or a vaginal birth after caesarean.

Text links

Chapter 39, 'Interventions in pregnancy, labour and birth' (Pairman et al., 2022).

A FINAL WORD

Decision making for women about mode of birth following a previous caesarean section is complex and requires supportive midwifery care (Davis et al., 2020). The rising rates of caesarean section indicate that more women will face decision making about the mode of birth for their next pregnancy. Midwives, therefore, play a pivotal role in counselling women about the mode of birth, including individualised discussions around benefits versus risks. It is important to think about the language that is used when working with women and to provide them with useful decision-making aids. Ultimately, it is the woman's decision, and the birth she chooses and her experience of birth will impact on her early mothering. Midwives need to work in collaborative practice with obstetricians when discussing the next birth after a caesarean section.

CHAPTER 18

Water immersion for labour and birth

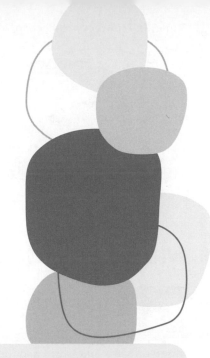

INTRODUCTION

This chapter introduces you to water immersion in labour and birth. Confidence facilitating water birth is a core skill for midwives as it is closely associated with physiological birth (Maude & Caplice in Pairman et al., 2022). This is supported by current evidence, which shows several important benefits surrounding maternal satisfaction. Clews et al. (2019) found that water birth gave women an enhanced sense of autonomy and control, and Ulfdottir (2018) found women valued the increased sense of privacy, safety, control and focus when giving birth in water. In addition, a Cochrane review in 2018 showed no evidence of increased adverse effects to the fetus/neonate or woman from labouring or giving birth in water and that water birth may reduce the number of women having an epidural (Cluett et al., 2018). Given that water birth provides choice for women, increases satisfaction and decreases intervention, skills and knowledge surrounding water birth remain an important area of education.

In this chapter we hear from Elise who is both a midwife and a mother. Elise gives her perspective on water immersion for labour and waterbirth from both of these perspectives.

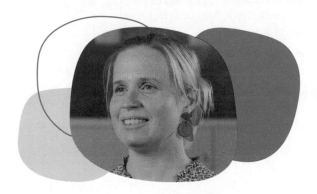

 View Elise's story or read the transcript.

Elise is a mother of two daughters. Elise chose to have her babies at home supported by a continuity of care model of midwifery care. She chose to use water immersion as a form of pain relief for labour with both of her births and ultimately birthed her babies into water. Elise shares her experience of water immersion and water birth and how important it was for her. Elise also offers some practical advice for labouring women considering water immersion and/or water birth and for attending midwives.

Birthing woman Elise's story

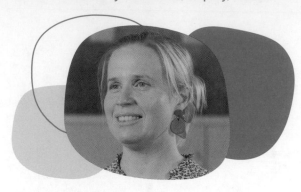

Midwife Elise's story

 View Elise's story or read the transcript.

Elise works as a midwife in a continuity of care group practice caseload midwifery model and provides care to women choosing to birth in a stand-alone birth centre or at home. She has vast experience supporting women who choose to use water immersion for labour and birth. Elise shares her tips and experiences of setting up for and supporting women choosing to use water immersion.

Reflection

1. What were the positive aspects of using water immersion during labour and birth from (the mother) Elise's perspective?

2. What enablers and barriers have you experienced or envisage for the use of water immersion in labour and/or water birth?

3. What benefits can you perceive from a midwives' perspective for water immersion in labour and water birth?

4. What concerns do you have as a midwife with regard to water immersion in labour and water birth?

5. What was Elise's main motivations for using water immersion in labour and ultimately having a water birth?

Inquiry

1. What clinical practice guidelines currently exist in your area regarding water immersion in labour/water birth? What are three reasons it may not be advisable for a woman to use water immersion?

2. Read Chapter 27 in Pairman et al. (2022). List three benefits of water birth for the woman, the baby and the midwife.

3. Read the 2018 Cochrane review (Cluett et al., 2018) on immersion in water during labour and birth: https://www.cochranelibrary.com/cdsr/doi/10.1002/14651858.CD000111.pub4/full and write down what you conclude from this review.

4. Read the article by Bovbjerg et al. (2021). List the maternal and neonatal outcomes the study reviewed. What is the conclusion of the study?

Action

1. You are providing care for Sam, a 23-year-old G1P0 in established labour. Sam asks to use the bath for pain relief but in your facility it is rarely used and in a separate room.

2. What barriers to using water immersion might Sam encounter? How would you address these?

3. What would you say to Sam about the safety of using water immersion for labour and possibly birth?

4. What equipment would you get ready given the bath is not in the birth room?

5. How would you support Sam in the bath?

6. Sam births in the bath and has a wonderful experience. Sam writes a letter to the hospital. What benefits do you think Sam would write about?

A FINAL WORD

The demand for water immersion in labour and water birth has increased over the past three decades with women wanting to find ways to naturally manage the pain of labour and midwives seeing water immersion as a non-pharmacological form of pain relief. Water immersion for labour and birth provides several important benefits for women with no evidence of increased adverse effects. Lack of skills and knowledge may contribute to a fear of water birth so by examining evidence, becoming aware of policies and practices in your facility, and by having a deep understanding of the benefits for women, midwives may feel better equipped to overcome barriers and support women in this choice.

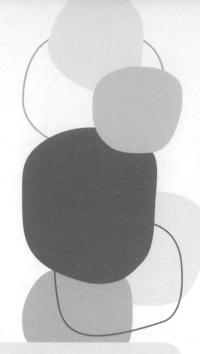

CHAPTER 19

Privately practising midwives

INTRODUCTION

Over a decade ago, consumer demand for homebirth was presented in a maternity services reform report (Dahlen et al., 2011). Publicly funded homebirth is limited in Australia despite evidence for improved outcomes (Homer et al., 2019). Many women, therefore, contract a privately practising endorsed midwife who provides homebirth services.

Endorsed midwives are required to meet the requirements of the Nursing and Midwifery Board of Australia and are qualified to prescribe scheduled medicines and provide associated services for midwifery practice in accordance with relevant state and territory legislation. To apply for endorsement, midwives are required to complete three years' full-time clinical practice (5000 hours) within six years of applying and complete an Australian Nursing and Midwifery Accreditation Council (ANMAC) approved program of study for prescribing medicines (Nursing and Midwifery Board of Australia, 2022). Endorsed midwives must also have professional indemnity insurance and be working in collaborative practice with an obstetrician or health service (Nursing and Midwifery Board of Australia, 2022).

Endorsed midwives must maintain a record of all midwifery practice, births and statistics related to birth as their records are audited from time to time by the registration authority.

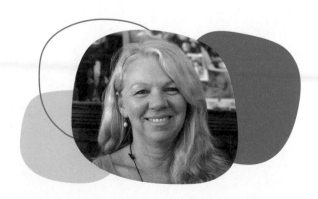

Sheryl's story

 View Sheryl's story or read the transcript.

Sheryl has been working as an independent midwife for more than 20 years. Working in private practice is described by Sheryl as a way of life, not a job. Sheryl describes herself as passionate about women and birth, stating that it makes a difference to the woman's birth outcome when she knows and trusts the midwife. Knowing the midwife provides the woman with one-to-one care throughout pregnancy, birth and the early postnatal period in a trusting relationship. Sheryl proposes that pregnancy and birth is a transformative process when a woman becomes a mother. During her 28 years of practice, Sheryl, along with other privately practising midwives, and consumers have been lobbying for more women to have access to homebirth.

Reflection

1. Sheryl says the most satisfying part of her work is the relationship she has with women and that when we look at her statistics, women choosing homebirth have a higher chance of having a normal birth. It is proposed that for women to birth normally they need to feel safe, nurtured, unobserved, cared for, important, valued, loved, trusted and, most importantly, relaxed (Sidery, 2014). The most appropriate environment would be in the comfort of her own home, surrounded by those who know and love her (Sidery, 2014). Think about the differences between the maternity service with which you are familiar and having a baby at home with a known midwife. How might working in midwifery continuity of care provide satisfaction to the midwife and address increasing staff attrition rates from standard maternity care practices?

2. Sheryl describes the midwife's role in pregnancy as preparing the woman to become a mother and the man to become a father. Sheryl says this is an ultimate transformation that she is privileged to be part of every day. Consider how a known midwife who provides midwifery care until 6 weeks postpartum in the woman's home will support the transition to parenthood.

Inquiry

1. List the requirements a midwife must achieve in order to be an endorsed midwife.

2. Privately practising midwives like Sheryl can apply for a Medicare provider number, making access to maternity care from a known and trusted midwife more affordable for many families. What must a midwife do in order to apply for a Medicare Provider number?

Action

1. Think about how you will work towards becoming an endorsed midwife. Develop a learning plan of what you will need to achieve once you have completed your program of study that leads to registration as a midwife in Australia. Your plan needs to include how you will achieve certain skills (e.g. perineal repair), where and how you will access education/experience for each skill and in what time frame.

2. Write a business plan as a privately practising midwifery business that will allow you to have a month's annual leave a year and back-up in the case of illness. Your business will need to generate enough income to support yourself in your current lifestyle and any dependants.

Text links

Chapters 1, 2, 3, 5 and 6 in *Midwifery Continuity of Care* (Homer et al., 2019).

A FINAL WORD

The evidence supports homebirth for women with an uncomplicated pregnancy with a qualified midwife networked into the health system. In addition, having a trusting relationship with a known midwife from continuity of care is beneficial to women and babies (Davis & Homer, 2016; Forster et al., 2016; Sandall et al., 2016). The challenge is for our maternity services—both public and private—to provide homebirth services to women and their families that choose their own midwife. As you work towards becoming an endorsed midwife, you will be meeting a growing demand for women wanting to access homebirth. As Sheryl says, 'I really do believe it is the best start for a family, to have a birth at home.'

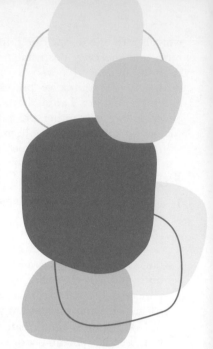

CHAPTER 20

Birthing a baby with a congenital anomaly— anencephaly

INTRODUCTION

Congenital anomalies occur in an estimated 6% of babies worldwide (World Health Organization (WHO), 2023). In Australia, the incidence of birth defects/congenital anomalies is lower than the global average, with 3% of babies born with a congenital anomaly in 2016 (Australian Institute of Health and Welfare (AIHW), 2022). Despite this lower rate, nearly one-third (31%) of perinatal deaths in Australia were caused by a congenital anomaly (AIHW, 2022), making this an important area of education for maternity care providers. The general causes of congenital anomalies include: unknown cause (50–60%), multifactorial inheritance (20–25%), chromosomal abnormalities (6–7%), mutant genes (7–8%) and environmental agents (7–10%) (Moore et al., 2016). Environmental factors include infection, pollution, nutritional deficiencies, illness and drug use (WHO, 2023), and socio-economic factors include maternal age and access to screening and healthcare.

Neural tube defects are the most common malformation of the central nervous system and arise from abnormalities during formation and closure of the neural tube. Anencephaly is a neural tube defect that occurs when the skull, scalp and brain of the fetus do not develop properly in utero. Approximately 1:5000–10,000 babies are born with anencephaly. Most pregnancies with anencephaly end in miscarriage or stillbirth, but babies born alive will usually only live for a few hours or days after birth (Moore et al., 2016).

This chapter discusses the birth of a baby with anencephaly from the perspective of a mother and a midwife caring for the birthing woman.

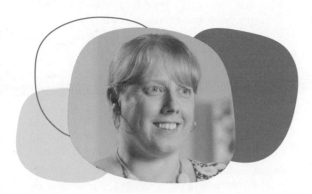

Vanessa's story

 View Vanessa's story or read the transcript.

Vanessa was pregnant with her second baby when at the 12-week ultrasound she was told her baby had anencephaly. Vanessa shares her story, including the process of making the decision to continue the pregnancy, the support she received from her midwife and other care providers and the experience of the birth of her son, Matthew.

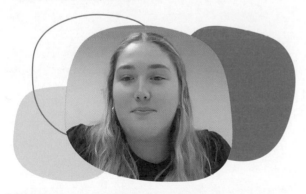

Ella's story

 View Ella's story or read the transcript.

Ella was a second year Bachelor of Midwifery student when she supported a woman to navigate the complex, confronting yet very private decision to carry her baby with anencephaly to term. In this story, Ella reflects on the comforting care she provided to the mother throughout her childbearing experience and shares some take-home messages from the perspective of a student.

Reflection

1. Vanessa recalls only having one significantly negative experience with a health professional during her pregnancy with Matthew. How do you think this experience could have been improved?

2. Vanessa was well supported throughout this pregnancy and birth by health professionals, family and friends. What do you think were some of the key factors that allowed Vanessa to receive such support? And what do you feel she valued the most?

3. Ella discusses the importance of a clear birth plan. Consider elements of care you might include in the same scenario. Why do you think this plan was important for the birthing mother?

4. Ella has several take-home messages that might help midwifery students in a similar scenario. Reflect on the support structures and services available to you and how you might practise self-care during challenging times as a student.

Inquiry

1. What are the main support services at your local facility to which you would refer a woman if she was found to be pregnant with a baby with anencephaly? Investigate whether genetic counselling and maternal fetal medicine are available to families in your area.

2. Visit the World Health Organization's information page for Congenital Disorders and explore the fact sheets. What are the most common severe birth defects?

3. How does the World Health Organization plan to promote primary prevention and improve the health of children with congenital anomalies? List five priority points.

Action

1. Make a resource that you could provide to women who are pregnant with and/or birthing a baby with a congenital abnormality.

2. Investigate the options surrounding postnatal care for women in your facility who have a baby with a congenital anomaly. Is there flexibility for rooming in, taking the baby home or family visits? Write a midwifery care plan including options for immediate and ongoing postnatal care for women with babies who have died from a known congenital anomaly.

3. The mother in Ella's story received her care from 'many different doctors'. Investigate whether there is a midwifery option of care for high-risk women in your facility and write a letter to your unit manager outlining the benefits of continuity of midwifery care in this scenario.

A FINAL WORD

The experience of carrying and birthing a baby with a congenital anomaly is an emotionally turbulent and challenging journey for the woman and her family. The midwife in Vanessa's story was able to support Vanessa and give her options for who else to speak to about her baby's diagnosis and help her in her decision-making processes. Ella, in her experience as a student midwife, also found that providing information about congenital anomalies and ensuring a clear plan for the pregnancy and birth was in place helped bring some feelings of control back to the family. As midwives, helping women to stay informed and being clear and transparent with options and information is one way to support families through the challenging experience of having a baby with a congenital anomaly.

CHAPTER 21

Cultural and linguistic diversity

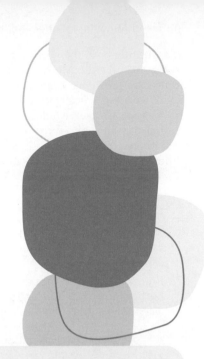

INTRODUCTION

Australia is a vibrant, multicultural country. Over 7 million people in Australia, comprising 27.6% of the population, were born overseas according to the latest census population data (ABS, 2022). The five most common overseas countries of birth are England, India, China, New Zealand and the Philippines. This rich, cultural diversity is one of Australia's greatest strengths, but with this diversity comes additional considerations when providing healthcare to culturally and/or linguistically diverse individuals. Racial discrimination and xenophobia are issues still prevalent within Australia (AHRC, 2014).

Midwives are in a unique position to provide maternity care to women from a variety of different ethnic and cultural backgrounds. Culture is defined as a group's own particular pattern or template for living and includes what a person thinks, says, does, believes and makes (Miller & Bear, 2019). Midwives need to demonstrate cultural safety in their practice, which is facilitated by open communication, understanding of diversity in worldviews and reflecting on their own culture and how it impacts on their healthcare practice. There can be specific cultural practices or preferences for women throughout pregnancy, labour and birth and the postpartum periods. Midwives need to be respectful of these cultural preferences, while still ensuring the delivery of safe care for the woman and her baby (Department of Health and Aged Care, 2020).

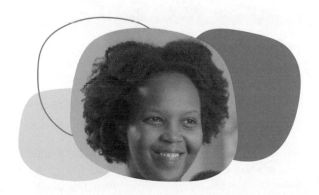

Emma's story

 View Emma's story or read the transcript.

Emma is a Burundi woman who migrated to Australia 17 years ago with her husband. Both of her children were born in Australia during the COVID-19 pandemic. Emma shares her experience of being a culturally diverse woman accessing maternity care, and outlines both the positive aspects of her care, as well as the prejudice she occasional experienced from healthcare providers. Emma describes how the post-natal period specifically is quite different in Australia from what women would experience in Burundi. Emma provides advice to those working in health-care to not make assumptions about people from different ethnic and cultural backgrounds when receiving maternity care.

Reflection

1. What were the positive aspects Emma experienced throughout her two pregnancy experiences?

2. Emma experienced both of her pregnancies and births during the COVID-19 pandemic. In what ways do you think the pandemic further impacted on women from culturally and linguistically diverse backgrounds when seeking maternity care?

3. Emma described the differences between the provision of postnatal care in Australia compared to her home country of Burundi. What were these differences and how can we support culturally diverse women in the postnatal time within the Australian healthcare system?

4. Women from culturally and linguistically diverse (CALD) backgrounds often have unique healthcare needs during the childbearing time. Social isolation, language barriers and different expectations surrounding pregnancy, birth and the postpartum period can make caring for CALD women more complex. What other supports or services do you think may be required when working with a woman from a culturally or linguistically diverse background?

Inquiry

1. Look at the latest AIHW Australia's Mothers and Babies report (2022) on maternal country of birth to learn about the diversity of women giving birth within Australia. Apart from Australia, which other countries of birth were most prevalent within the statistics? https://www.aihw.gov.au/reports/mothers-babies/australias-mothers-babies/contents/demographics-of-mothers-and-babies/maternal-country-of-birth

2. Consider how we can support women with limited English throughout their childbearing experience. Locate your local state or facility guideline on the use of healthcare interpreters for people who speak languages other than

English. In what ways could an interpreter assist a woman throughout her childbearing journey?

3. Does being a woman from a culturally diverse background increase the risks of adverse outcomes for the mother and the baby? Research this issue and list the main risks you find.

4. Midwives need to establish trusting and non-discriminatory relationships with all women in their care. Which of the standards in the NMBA Midwife Standards for Practice (2018) relate to the provision of midwifery care for culturally diverse women?

Action

1. Browse through some of the pregnancy and postnatal leaflets available in different languages from the website below. You may choose to use these when providing midwifery care to women and families who are from a CALD background. http://www.mhcs.health.nsw.gov.au/publicationsandresources#c3=eng&b_start=0&c1=Pregnancy±and±post±natal

2. Investigate what culturally diverse support groups are available in your area. Find the contact details and when and where group meetings are held.

3. Read the article by Hogan et al. (2018) and consider the importance of cultural empathy in your midwifery practice.

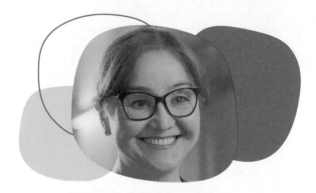

Sabera's story

 View Sabera's story or read the transcript.

Sabera is an Afghan midwife who migrated to Australia as a refugee. Sabera completed a PhD investigating women's views of care provided during pregnancy to those who have undergone female genital mutilation (FGM) overseas. Sabera shares her thoughts on why her research is important and the key findings, including tips to midwives to provide evidence-based and holistic care.

Reflection

1. Women from CALD backgrounds often have unique customs, traditions and religious practices. Some of these practices impact their health, such as FGM. What other supports or services do you think may be required when working with a woman who has experienced FGM?

2. Consider your culture and reflect on practices that might differ from others. How does your unconscious bias impact on how you care for those who have different cultural backgrounds from you?

Inquiry

1. Look at the latest Australian Institute of Health and Welfare (2019) data and the prevalence estimates for FGM/cutting: https://www.aihw.gov.au/getmedia/f210a1d8-5a3a-4336-80c5-ca6bdc2906d5/aihw-phe-230.pdf.aspx?inline=true. Are you surprised by the prevalence estimates?

2. Using the same source as above from the AIHW (2019), investigate which countries have FGM/C-practising communities and the areas where these women live in Australia. Do you feel it is likely you will provide care for a woman in your midwifery career who has undergone FGM/C?

Action

1. Identify services and resources available in your area that support women who have undergone FGM/C.

2. Review and undertake training, such as from the National Education Toolkit for Female Genital Mutilation/Cutting Awareness (NETFA) https://netfa.com.au/ or PLAN https://www.plan.org.au/why-girls/our-work/ending-female-genital-mutilation-fgm/.

3. Read the statement developed by the Royal Australian and New Zealand College of Obstetricians and Gynaecologists (RANZCOG) https://ranzcog.edu.au/wp-content/uploads/2022/05/Female-Genital-Mutilation-FGM.pdf and complete the online modules available.

A FINAL WORD

Australia is a multicultural country with the number of people born overseas continuing to rise. As such, midwives will encounter a variety of women from different ethnic and cultural backgrounds within their practice. Both student midwives and registered midwives must practise in a way that is culturally safe and appropriate for women and their families and be respectful of the unique cultural needs and preferences of women. Midwives must ensure culturally diverse women are well supported throughout their childbearing experience, which may at times require the involvement of interpreter services.

CHAPTER 22

Working with a woman with physical and/or intellectual disabilities

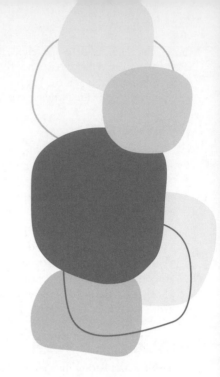

INTRODUCTION

Women with disabilities make up approximately 9–10% of birthing women in Australia and globally (Malouf et al., 2017; Smithson et al., 2021). Disabilities come in many forms, including physical, sensory and intellectual, and are not always easily perceived by midwives and other health professionals. Women with disabilities have many vulnerabilities, in addition to the complexity of their disability, and often have mental health comorbidities. Despite this, women with disabilities do not feature as a specific vulnerable group in policy documents, which in turn exacerbates barriers to maternity care and influences outcomes for their success (Williams, 2021). As such, many women with disabilities may have unmet needs when receiving maternity care as there is often limited knowledge among midwives as to how to meet the unique needs of these women (Pituch et al., 2022).

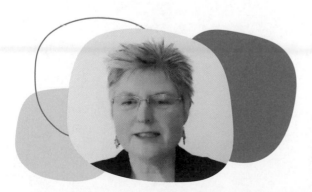

Namira's story

 View Namira's story or read the transcript.

In this video, Namira discusses her own experience as a midwife, and as a mum, of supporting and advocating for people with a disability. Namira discusses thinking about disability from the person's perspective and the importance of listening and flexible practice. Namira then gives an example of what listening and working to a person's strengths can achieve.

Reflection

1. In her discussion, Namira talks about how people view their disability and how significant they consider it to be. When working with a mother with a disability, how might you communicate with her, and support her to resonate with her view?

2. When discussing prenatal screening with parents with a disability, what considerations would you include in this discussion?

3. Namira discusses the importance of provider attitudes affecting the support for mothers with disabilities to transition to motherhood. Consider your own interactions with people with disabilities (not necessarily a woman or adult)— how did you feel? How did you interact, and how might your actions be perceived by the person with a disability?

Inquiry

1. Namira's discussion of factors that can contribute to outcomes for mothers with disabilities included hospital policies, provider attitudes and available resources. Which of the NMBA Midwife Standards for Practice (2018) can you link to disability maternity care?

2. Disclosure of disability can contribute to barriers in maternity care. Read 'How are women with a disability identified in maternity services in Australia? A cross-sectional survey of maternity managers' by Benzie et al. (2022). What did their research find, and how might this affect ongoing care for this group of women?

3. How does the World Health Organization define disability, and how is this different from the medical model of disability care?

4. The terms 'visible' and 'invisible' in relation to disabilities are often used—what is meant by each, and provide examples of both disabilities.

5. What is meant by the term 'disenfranchised grief' and how does this relate to mothers with a disability?

6. What services are available in your local area that could assist women with disabilities during pregnancy, birth and early parenting? (These could be local services, or online services and resources.)

Action

You are providing care in the postnatal ward to a mother with an intellectual disability. Child protection services were involved in her care just prior to the birth and there is a question about whether she should take her baby home. She is reluctant to talk with staff, and is seen as non-compliant.

1. Consider why she might be uncommunicative, and write down some strategies for working with this mother.

2. What resources could you provide to her to assist her in developing her parenting skills?

3. How could you better advocate for her?

4. Write down a list of other providers/ professionals with whom you might consult who could advocate for this mother to take her baby home.

5. What could have been done in pregnancy to ensure this mother was well set up to succeed?

6. If the decision was made for the baby to go into foster or kinship care, what steps could you take to make this a less traumatic experience for her?

A FINAL WORD

Becoming a parent is an aspiration for many people within the community. The saying 'it takes a village to raise a child' has been supported over the past decade by evidence-based research. Despite this, people with disabilities still find they are not supported in becoming parents, and can be actively discouraged from pursuing this choice in their lives. Namira has provided some strategies to assist providers, and especially midwives, to work with these mothers: listen to them, see their disability from their point of view and find ways to work around the barriers through accessing resources and advocacy. Most importantly, setting women up to succeed from early pregnancy, and how you might make the transition to motherhood a positive one, even when child protection services are involved. It is important to remember and acknowledge the woman's role as 'mother' even when she does not care for the baby every day. She will always be known as 'mother' to that child.

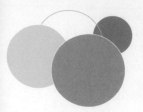

Further readings and references

Chapter 1

Australian Nursing and Midwifery Accreditation Council. (2021). *Midwife Accreditation Standards 2021.* Australian Nursing and Midwifery Council. https://www.anmac.org.au/standards-and-review/midwife.

Baird, K., Hastie, C. R., Stanton, P., & Gamble, J. (2021). Learning to be a midwife: Midwifery students' experiences of an extended placement within a midwifery group practice. *Women and Birth*. https://doi.org/10.1016/j.wombi.2021.01.002.

Beggs, B., Koshy, L., & Neiterman, E. (2021). Women's perceptions and experiences of breastfeeding: A scoping review of the literature. *BMC Public Health, 21*(1), 2169. https://doi.org/10.1186/s12889-021-12216-3.

Bradford, B. F., Wilson, A. N., Portela, A., McConville, F., Fernandez Turienzo, C., & Homer, C. S. E. (2022). Midwifery continuity of care: A scoping review of where, how, by whom and for whom? *PLOS Global Public Health, 2*(10), Article e0000935. https://doi.org/10.1371/journal.pgph.0000935.

Browne, J., & Taylor, J. (2014). It's a good thing…': Women's views on their continuity experiences with midwifery students from one Australian region. *Midwifery, 30*(3), e108–e114. https://doi.org/10.1016/j.midw.2013.11.006.

Carter, A. G., Wilkes, E., Gamble, J., Sidebotham, M., & Creedy, D. K. (2015). Midwifery students' experiences of an innovative clinical placement model embedded within midwifery continuity of care in Australia. *Midwifery, 31*(8), 765–771. https://doi.org/10.1016/j.midw.2015.04.006.

Catling, C., Rossiter, C., Cummins, A., & McIntyre, E. (2022). Midwifery workplace culture in Sydney, Australia. *Women and Birth: Journal of the Australian College of Midwives, 35*(4), e379–e388. https://doi.org/10.1016/j.wombi.2021.07.001.

COAG Health Council. (2019). *Woman-centred care: Strategic directions for Australian maternity services.* Canberra: COAG Health Council.

Cummins, A. M., Catling, C., & Homer, C. S. E. (2018). Enabling new graduate midwives to work in midwifery continuity of care models: A conceptual model for implementation. *Women and Birth, 31*(5), 343–349. https://doi.org/10.1016/j.wombi.2017.11.007.

Cummins, A. M., Denney-Wilson, E., & Homer, C. S. E. (2015). The experiences of new graduate midwives working in midwifery continuity of care models in Australia. *Midwifery, 31*(4), 438–444. https://doi.org/10.1016/j.midw.2014.12.013.

Ferguson, B., Capper, T., Brookfield, J., Williamson, M., & Lovegrove, M. (2018). Benefits of continuity models of care in building mutual support and nurturing between women and midwifery students. Does continuity of care foster clinical confidence, emotional resilience and influence career goals? *Women and Birth: Journal of the Australian College of Midwives, 31*, S9–S10. https://doi.org/10.1016/j.wombi.2018.08.037.

Forster, D. A., McLachlan, H. L., Davey, M. A., Biro, M. A., Farrell, T., Gold, L., Flood, M., Shafiei, T., & Waldenström, U. (2016). Continuity of care by a primary midwife (caseload midwifery) increases women's satisfaction with antenatal, intrapartum and postpartum care: Results from the COSMOS randomised controlled trial. *BMC Pregnancy Childbirth, 16*, 28. https://doi.org/10.1186/s12884-016-0798-y.

Homer, C., Leap, N., Brodie, P., & Sandall, J. (2019). *Midwifery continuity of care* (2nd ed.). Elsevier.

International Confederation of Midwives. (2021). *ICM Global Standards for Midwifery Education*. https://www.internationalmidwives.org/assets/files/general-files/2021/09/global-standards-for-midwifery-education_2021_en.pdf

McLachlan, H., Forster, D., Davey, M.-A., Farrell, T., Gold, L., Biro, M., Albers, L., Flood, M., Oats, J., & Waldenström, U. (2012). Effects of continuity of care by a primary midwife (caseload midwifery) on caesarean section rates in women of low obstetric risk: The COSMOS randomised controlled trial. *BJOG: An International Journal of Obstetrics & Gynaecology, 119*(12), 1483–1492.

Medley, N., Vogel, J. P., Care, A., & Alfirevic, Z. (2018). Interventions during pregnancy to prevent preterm birth: An overview of Cochrane systematic reviews. *Cochrane Database of Systematic Reviews*(11). https://doi.org/10.1002/14651858.CD012505.pub2.

Mortensen, B., Diep, L. M., Lukasse, M., Lieng, M., Dwekat, I., Elias, D., & Fosse, E. (2019). Women's satisfaction with midwife-led continuity of care: An observational study in Palestine. *BMJ Open, 9*(11). 10.1136/bmjopen-2019-030324.

Newton, M. S., McLachlan, H. L., Willis, K. F., & Forster, D. A. (2014). Comparing satisfaction and burnout between caseload and standard care midwives: Findings from two cross-sectional surveys conducted in Victoria, Australia. *BMC Pregnancy and Childbirth, 14*(1), 426.

Nursing and Midwifery Board of Australia. (2018). *Midwife standards for practice*. file:///C:/Users/034761/Downloads/Nursing-and-Midwifery-Board—Professional-standards—Advance-copy—Midwife-standards-for-practice—Effective-1-October-2018%20(7).PDF

Pairman, S., Tracy, S. K., Dahlen, H., & Dixon, S. (2022). *Midwifery: Preparation for Practice* (5th ed.). Elsevier.

Sandall, J., Soltani, H., Gates, S., Shennan, A., & Devane, D. (2016). Midwife-led continuity models versus other models of care for childbearing women. *Cochrane Database of Systematic Reviews*(4), Article CD004667. https://doi.org/10.1002/14651858.CD004667.

Sidebotham, M., & Fenwick, J. (2019). Midwifery students' experiences of working within a midwifery caseload model. *Midwifery, 74*, 21–28. https://doi.org/10.1016/j.midw.2019.03.008.

Stulz, V., Elmir, D. R., & Reilly, H. (2020). Evaluation of a student-led midwifery group practice: A woman's perspective. *Midwifery, 86*, Article 102691. https://doi.org/10.1016/j.midw.2020.102691.

World Health Organization. (2018). *Preterm birth*. World Health Organization. https://www.who.int/news-room/fact-sheets/detail/preterm-birth

Chapter 2

Australian College of Midwives (ACM). (2021). *National Midwifery Guidelines for Consultation and Referral*. ACM.

Australian Institute of Health Welfare. (2022). Australia's mothers and babies. https://www.aihw.gov.au/reports/mothers-babies/australias-mothers-babies

Bohren, M. A., Hofmeyr, G. J., Sakala, C., Fukuzawa, R. K., & Cuthbert, A. (2017). Continuous support for women during childbirth. *Cochrane Database of Systematic Reviews*(7). https://doi.org/10.1002/14651858.CD003766.pub6.

Brocklehurst, P., Hardy, P., Hollowell, J., Linsell, L., Macfarlane, A., McCourt, C., Marlow, N., Miller, A., Newburn, M., Petrou, S., Puddicombe, D., Redshaw, M., Rowe, R., Sandall, J., Silverton, L., Stewart, M., & Birthplace in England Collaborative Group. (2011). Perinatal and maternal outcomes by planned place of birth for healthy women with low risk pregnancies: The Birthplace in England national prospective cohort study. *BMJ, 343*(7840), 243. 377;751;256;554;1177;2265;1933;1407;1483;-1117. https://doi.org/10.1136/bmj.d7400.

Catling, C. (2020). *National publicly-funded homebirth*. Sydney: University of Technology. https://www.uts.edu.au/research-and-teaching/our-research/centre-midwifery-child-and-family-health/research/past-projects/national-publicly-funded-homebirth.

Dahlen, H., Jackson, M., Schmied, V., Tracy, S., & Priddis, H. (2011). Birth centres and the national maternity services review: Response to consumer demand or compromise? *Women and Birth, 24*(4), 165–172. https://doi.org/10.1016/j.wombi.2010.11.001.

Davis, D., Baddock, S., Pairman, S., Hunter, M., Benn, C., Wilson, D., Dixon, L., & Herbison, P. (2011). Planned place of birth in New Zealand: Does it affect mode of birth and intervention rates among low-risk women? *Birth, 38*(2), 111–119. https://doi.org/10.1111/j.1523-536X.2010.00458.x.

de Jonge, A., van der Goes, B. Y., Ravelli, A. C. J., Amelink-Verburg, M. P., Mol, B. W., Nijhuis, J. G., Bennebroek Gravenhorst, J., & Buitendijk, S. E. (2009). Perinatal mortality and morbidity in a nationwide cohort of 529,688 low-risk planned home and hospital births. *BJOG: An International Journal of Obstetrics and Gynaecology, 116*(9), 1177–1184. https://doi.org/10.1111/j.1471-0528.2009.02175.x.

Homer, C. S. E., Cheah, S. L., Rossiter, C., Dahlen, H. G., Ellwood, D., Foureur, M. J., Forster, D. A., McLachlan, H. L., Oats, J. J. N., Sibbritt, D., Thornton, C., & Scarf, V. L. (2019). Maternal and perinatal outcomes by planned place of birth in Australia 2000 –2012: A linked population data study. *BMJ Open, 9*(10). https://doi.org/10.1136/bmjopen-2019-029192.

Homer, C. S. E., Davies-Tuck, M., Dahlen, H. G., & Scarf, V. L. (2021). The impact of planning for COVID-19 on private practising midwives in Australia. *Women and Birth: Journal of the Australian College of Midwives, 34*(1), e32–e37. https://doi.org/10.1016/j.wombi.2020.09.013.

Hutton, E. K., Reitsma, A., Simioni, J., Brunton, G., & Kaufman, K. (2019). Perinatal or neonatal mortality among women who intend at the onset of labour to give birth at home compared to women of low obstetrical risk who intend to give birth in hospital: A systematic review and meta-analyses. *EClinicalMedicine, 14*, 59–70. https://doi.org/10.1016/j.eclinm.2019.07.005.

Kluwgant, D., Homer, C., & Dahlen, H. (2022). 'Never let a good crisis go to waste': Positives from disrupted maternity care in Australia during COVID-19. *Midwifery, 110*, Article 103340. https://doi.org/10.1016/j.midw.2022.103340.

Lindgren, H., & Erlandsson, K. (2011). She leads, he follows – fathers' experiences of a planned home birth: A Swedish interview study. *Sexual & Reproductive Healthcare, 2*(2), 65–70. https://doi.org/10.1016/j.srhc.2010.12.002.

Pairman, S., Tracy, S. K., Dahlen, H., & Dixon, S. (2022). *Midwifery: Preparation for Practice* (5th ed.). Elsevier.

Sweeney, S., & O'Connell, R. (2015). Puts the magic back into life: Fathers' experience of planned home birth. *Women and Birth: Journal of the Australian College of Midwives, 28*(2), 148–153. https://doi.org/10.1016/j.wombi.2014.12.001.

World Health Organization. (2023). Breastfeeding. https://www.who.int/health-topics/breastfeeding#tab=tab_1

Chapter 3

Hannah, M. E., Hannah, W. J., Hewson, S. A., Hodnett, E. D., Saigal, S., & Willan, A. R. (2000). Planned caesarean section versus planned vaginal birth for breech presentation at term: A randomised multicentre trial. *Lancet, 356*(9239), 1375–1383.

Marshall, J. E., & Raynor, M. D. (Eds.). (2020). *Myles textbook for midwives* (17th ed.). Elsevier.

Nursing and Midwifery Board of Australia (NMBA). (2018). *National competency standards for the midwife*. https://www.nursingmidwiferyboard.gov.au/Codes-Guidelines-Statements/Professional-standards/Midwife-standards-for-practice.aspx

Royal Australian and New Zealand College of Obstetricians and Gynaecologists. (2021). Management of breech presentation. https://ranzcog.edu.au/wp-content/uploads/2022/05/Management-of-breech-presentation.pdf

FURTHER READING

Pairman, S., Tracy, S. K., Dahlen, H., & Dixon, S. (2022). *Midwifery: Preparation for Practice* (5th ed.). Elsevier.

WEBSITE

https://ranzcog.edu.au/wp-content/uploads/2022/06/Breech-presentation-at-the-end-of-your-pregnancy.pdf

Chapter 4

Aitken, R. J. (2022). The changing tide of human fertility. *Human Reproduction, 37*(4), 629–638. https://doi.org/10.1093/humrep/deac011.

Australian Government, Department of Health and Aged Care. (2020). *Clinical practice guidelines.* https://www.health.gov.au/resources/pregnancy-care-guidelines

Charalambous, C., Webster, A., & Schuh, M. (2023). Aneuploidy in mammalian oocytes and the impact of maternal ageing. *Nature Reviews Molecular Cell Biology, 24*(1), 27–44. https://doi.org/10.1038/s41580-022-00517-3.

Seshadri, S., Morris, G., Serhal, P., & Saab, W. (2021). Assisted conception in women of advanced maternal age. *Best Practice & Research: Clinical Obstetrics & Gynaecology, 70*, 10–20. https://doi.org/10.1016/j.bpobgyn.2020.06.012.

FURTHER READING

Pairman, S., Tracy, S. K., Dahlen, H., & Dixon, S. (2022). *Midwifery: Preparation for Practice* (5th ed.). Elsevier.

Chapter 5

Al-Shaikh, G. K., Ibrahim, G. H., Fayed, A. A., & Al-Mandeel, H. (2017). Grand multiparity and the possible risk of adverse maternal and neonatal outcomes: A dilemma to be deciphered. *BMC Pregnancy and Childbirth, 17*(310). https://doi.org/10.1186/s12884-017-1508-0.

Hochler, H., Wainstock, T., Lipschuetz, M., Sheiner, E., Ezra, Y., Yagel, S., & Walfisch, A. (2020). Grandmultiparity, maternal age, and the risk for uterine rupture—A multicenter cohort study. *Acta Obstetricia Gynecologica Scandinavica, 99*(2), 267–273. https://doi.org/10.1111/aogs.13725.

Muniro, Z., Tarimo, C. S., Mahande, M. J., Maro, E., & Mchome, B. (2019). Grand multiparity as a predictor of adverse pregnancy outcome among women who delivered at a tertiary hospital in Northern Tanzania. *BMC Pregnancy and Childbirth, 19*(222). https://doi.org/10.1186/s12884-019-2377-5.

Nursing and Midwifery Board Ahpra (NMBA). (2018). *Code of Conduct for Midwives.*,https://www.nursingmidwiferyboard.gov.au/codes-guidelines-statements/professional-standards.aspx

FURTHER READING

Pairman, S., Tracy, S. K., Dahlen, H., & Dixon, S. (2022). *Midwifery: Preparation for Practice* (5th ed.). Elsevier.

Chapter 6

Australian Institute of Health and Welfare (AIHW). (2021). Australia's mothers and babies: maternal deaths. https://www.aihw.gov.au/reports/mothers-babies/maternal-deaths-australia

Australian Institute of Health and Welfare (AIHW). (2022). *Rural and remote health.* https://www.aihw.gov.au/reports/australias-health/rural-and-remote-health

Council of Australian Governments Health Council. (2019). *Woman-centred care: Strategic directions for Australian maternity services.* Australian Government: Department of Health and Aged Care. https://www.health.gov.au/resources/publications/woman-centred-care-strategic-directions-for-australian-maternity-services.

FURTHER READING

Pairman, S., Tracy, S. K., Dahlen, H., & Dixon, S. (2022). *Midwifery: Preparation for Practice* (5th ed.). Elsevier.

Rolfe, M., Donoghue, D. A., Longman, J. M., Pilcher, J., Kildea, S., Kruske, S., Kornelsen, J., Grzybowski, S., Barclay, L., & Morgan, G. G. (2017). The distribution of maternity services across rural and remote Australia: Does it reflect population need? *BMC Health Services Research, 17*(163), 1–13. https://bmchealthservres.biomedcentral.com/articles/10.1186/s12913-017-2084-8.

Chapter 7

Australian College of Midwives. (2021). *National Midwifery Guidelines for Consultation and Referral* (4th ed). https://midwives.org.au/Web/Web/About-ACM/Guideline-Statements.aspx.

Australian Institute of Health and Welfare (AIHW). (2021). *Australia's mothers and babies*. Cat. no. PER 101. https://www.aihw.gov.au/reports/mothers-babies/australias-mothers-babies/contents/about

Betran, A., Ye, J., Moller, A., Zhang, J., Gülmezoglu, A., & Torloni, M. (2016). The increasing trend in caesarean section rates: Global, regional and national estimates: 1990–2014. *Public Library of Science, 11*(2), Article e0148343.

Hanahoe, M. (2020). Midwifery-led care can lower caesarean section rates according to the Robson ten group classification system. *European Journal of Midwifery, 4*, 7.

Mapp, T., & Hudson, K. G. (2005a). Feelings and fears during obstetric emergencies—1. *The British Journal of Midwifery, 13*(1), 30–35.

Marshall, J. E, & Raynor, M. D. (2020). *Myles Textbook for Midwives* (17th ed.). Elsevier.

Mapp, T., & Hudson, K. (2005b). Feelings and fears during obstetric emergencies—2. *The British Journal of Midwifery, 13*(1), 36–40.

NSW Health. (2010). *Maternity: Towards normal birth in NSW*. NSW Department of Health.

NSW Health. (2014). *Maternity—Supporting women in their next birth after caesarean section*. NBAC. https://www1.health.nsw.gov.au/pds/ActivePDSDocuments/GL2014_004.pdf.

Nursing and Midwifery Board of Australia (NMBA). (2018). *Midwife standards for practice*. https://www.nursingmidwiferyboard.gov.au/codes-guidelines-statements/professional-standards.aspx

Pairman, S., Tracy, S. K., Dahlen, H., & Dixon, S. (2022). *Midwifery: Preparation for Practice* (5th ed.). Elsevier.

World Health Organization (WHO). (2018). WHO recommendations: Non-clinical interventions to reduce unnecessary caesarean sections. https://www.who.int/publications/i/item/9789241550338

Chapter 8

Australian Bureau of Statistics (ABS). (2018). *Same-sex couples in Australia, 2016*. https://www.abs.gov.au/ausstats/abs@.nsf/Lookup/2071.0main+features852016

Crouch, S. R., Waters, E., McNair, R., & Power, J. (2014a). The health perspectives of Australian adolescents from same-sex parent families: A mixed methods study. *Child: Care, Health and Development, 41*(3), 356–364. https://doi.org/10.1111/cch.12180.

Crouch, S. R., Waters, E., McNair, R., Power, J., & Davis, E. (2014b). Parent-reported measures of child health and wellbeing in same-sex parent families: A cross sectional survey. *BMC Public Health, 14*, 635. https://doi.org/10.1186/1471-2458-14-635.

Department of Social Services. (2020). *Recognition of same-sex relationships*. Australian Government. https://www.dss.gov.au/our-responsibilities/families-and-children/programs-services/recognition-of-same-sex-relationships#:~:text=From%201%20July%202009%20changes,%2C%20as%20opposite%2Dsex%20couples.

Hammond, C. (2014). Exploring same sex couples' experiences of maternity care. *British Journal of Midwifery, 22*(7), 1–7. https://doi.org/10.12968/bjom.2014.22.7.495.

Mazrekaj, D., De Witte, K., & Cabus, S. (2020). School outcomes of children raised by same-sex parents: Evidence from administrative panel data. *American Sociological Review, 85*(5), 830–856. https://doi.org/10.1177/0003122420957249.

Mazrekaj, D., Fischer, M. M., & Bos, H. M. W. (2022). Behavioral outcomes of children with same-sex parents in The Netherlands. *International Journal of Environmental Research and Public Health, 19*(10), 5922. https://doi.org/10.3390/ijerph19105922.

Nursing and Midwifery Board of Australia (NMBA). (2018) *Midwife standards for practice*. https://www.nursingmidwiferyboard.gov.au/Codes-Guidelines-Statements/Professional-standards.aspx

Stewart, K., & O'Reilly, P. (2017). Exploring the attitudes, knowledge and beliefs of nurses and midwives of the healthcare needs of the LGBTQ population: An integrative review. *Nurse Education Today, 53*, 67–77. https://doi.org/10.1016/j.nedt.2017.04.008.

Soled, K. R. S., Niles, P. M., Mantell, E., Dansky, M., Bockting, W., & George, M (2022). Childbearing at the margins: A systematic metasynthesis of sexual and gender diverse childbearing experiences. *Birth Issues in Perinatal Care*. [in press]. https://doi.org/10.1111/birt.12678.

FURTHER READING

Attorney-General's Office. (2019). *Marriage equality in Australia.* Australian Government. https://www.ag.gov.au/families-and-marriage/marriage/marriage-equality-australia

Australian Human Rights Commission. (2007). *Same-sex: Same entitlements report. Chapter 5.* Sydney: AHRC. https://www.humanrights.gov.au/publications/same-sex-same-entitlements-chapter-5#2.

Australian Institute of Family Studies. (2020). *Families then and now: Couple relationships.* Australian Government. https://aifs.gov.au/research/research-reports/families-then-now-couple-relationships.

Chapman, R., Wardrop, J., Zappia, T., Watkins, R., & Shields, L. (2012). The experiences of Australian lesbian couples becoming parents: Deciding, searching and birthing. *Journal of Clinical Nursing, 21*(13–14), 1878–1885. https://doi.org/10.1111/j.1365-2702.2011.04007.x.

Pairman, S., Tracy, S. K., Dahlen, H., & Dixon, S. (2022). *Midwifery: Preparation for Practice* (5th ed.). Elsevier.

Qu, L. (2020). *Couple relationships.* Australian Government: Australian Institute of Family Studies. https://aifs.gov.au/sites/default/files/2022-07/2007_AFTN_Couples_update2022.pdf.

Chapter 9

Australian Institute of Family Studies. (2010). *Supporting young parents.* https://aifs.gov.au/resources/practice-guides/supporting-young-parents

Australian Institute of Health and Welfare (AIHW). (2022). *Australia's children: Teenage mothers.* https://www.aihw.gov.au/reports/children-youth/australias-children/contents/health/teenage-mothers

Karai, A., Gyurkovits, Z., András Nyári, T., Sári, T., Németh, G., & Orvos, H. (2019). Adverse perinatal outcome in teenage pregnancies: An analysis of a 5-year period in Southeastern Hungary. *The Journal of Maternal-Fetal and Neonatal Medicine, 32*(14), 2376–2379. https://doi.org/10.1080/14767058.2018.1438393.

Mohammed Arshadh, N. S., & Tengku Muda, T. E. A. (2020). A review of social acceptance, psychosocial implications and coping mechanisms of teenage mothers. *International Journal of Social Science Research, 2*(1), 1–12. https://myjms.mohe.gov.my/index.php/ijssr/article/view/8284/5289.

Nolan, S., & Hendricks, J. (2019). Care for pregnant and parenting adolescents. In E. Jefford, & J. Jomeen (Eds.), *Empowering decision-making in midwifery: A global perspective* (1st ed.). Routledge.

Pinho-Popeu, M., Sutia, F. G., Pastore, D. A., Palino, D. S. M., & Pinto e Silva, J. L. (2017). Anemia in pregnant adolescents: Impact of treatment on perinatal outcomes. *Journal of Maternal-Fetal and Neonatal Medicine, 30*(10), 1158–1162. https://doi.org/10.1080/14767058.2016.1205032.

FURTHER READING

Marino, J. L., Lewis, L. N., Bateson, D., Hickey, M., & Skinner, S. R. (2016). Teenage mothers. *Australian Family Physician, 45*(10), 712–717. https://www.racgp.org.au/afp/2016/october/teenage-mothers/.

Pairman, S., Tracy, S. K., Dahlen, H., & Dixon, S. (2022). *Midwifery: Preparation for Practice* (5th ed.). Elsevier.

Chapter 10

Australian Institute of Health and Welfare (AIHW). (2022). *Indigenous health and wellbeing.* https://www.aihw.gov.au/reports/australias-health/indigenous-health-and-wellbeing

Bainbridge, R., McCalman, J., Clifford, A., & Tsey, K. (for the Closing the Gap Clearinghouse). (2015). *Cultural competency in the delivery of health services for Indigenous people.* AIHW.

Commonwealth of Australia. (2022). *Commonwealth closing the gap annual report 2022.* https://www.niaa.gov.au/sites/default/files/publications/niaa-closing-the-gap-annual-report-2022.pdf

Nursing and Midwifery Board of Australia (NMBA). (2018). *Midwife standards for practice.* https://www.nursingmidwiferyboard.gov.au/Codes-Guidelines-Statements/Professional-standards/Midwife-standards-for-practice.aspx

International Confederation of Midwives. (2014). *Code of Ethics for Midwives.* https://www.internationalmidwives.org/assets/files/general-files/2019/10/eng-international-code-of-ethics-for-midwives.pdf

FURTHER READING

Pairman, S., Tracy, S. K., Dahlen, H., & Dixon, S. (2022). *Midwifery: Preparation for Practice* (5th ed.). Elsevier.

Chapter 11

Allport, B. S., Johnson, S., Aqil, A., Labrique, A. B., Nelson, T., KC, A., Carabas, Y., & Marcell, A. V. (2018). Promoting father involvement for child and family health. *Academic Pediatrics, 18*(7), 746–753. https://doi.org/10.1016/j.acap.2018.03.011.

Jessee, V., & Adamsons, K. (2018). Father involvement and father–child relationship quality: An intergenerational perspective. *Parenting, Science and Practice, 18*(1), 28–44. https://doi.org/10.1080/15295192.2018.1405700.

FURTHER READING

Al Namir, H. M. A., Brady, A.-M., & Gallagher, L (2017). Fathers and breastfeeding: Attitudes, involvement and support. *British Journal of Midwifery, 25*(7), 426–440. https://doi.org/10.12968/bjom.2017.25.7.426.

Mahesh, P. K. B., Gunathunga, M. W., Arnold, S. M., Jayasinghe, C., Pathirana, S., Makarim, M. F., Manawadu, P. M., & Senanayake, S. J. (2018). Effectiveness of targeting fathers for breastfeeding promotion: systematic review and meta-analysis. *BMC Public Health, 18*(1), 1140. https://doi.org/10.1186/s12889-018-6037-x.

Pairman, S., Tracy, S. K., Dahlen, H., & Dixon, S. (2022). *Midwifery: Preparation for Practice* (5th ed.). Elsevier.

Chapter 12

Australian Institute of Health and Welfare, 2022

Macdonald, S., & Johnson, G. (Eds.). (2017). *Mayes' midwifery* (15th ed.). Elsevier.

Nursing and Midwifery Board of Australia (NMBA). (2018). Code of conduct for midwives. https://www.nursingmidwiferyboard.gov.au/Codes-Guidelines-Statements/Professional-standards.aspx

Skinner, J., & Maude, R. (2016). The tensions of uncertainty: Midwives managing risk in and of their practice. *Midwifery, 38*, 35–41. https://doi.org/10.1016/j.midw.2016.03.006.

FURTHER READING

Pairman, S., Tracy, S. K., Dahlen, H., & Dixon, S. (2022). *Midwifery: Preparation for Practice* (5th ed.). Elsevier.

Chapter 13

Australian College of Midwives. (2021). *National Midwifery Guidelines for Consultation and Referral* (4th ed). https://midwives.org.au/Web/Web/About-ACM/Guideline-Statements.aspx.

Australian Institute of Health and Welfare (AIHW). (2022). *Maternal deaths.* https://www.aihw.gov.au/reports/mothers-babies/maternal-deaths-australia

American Sociological Association. (2014, 18 August). *'Super-Parent' cultural pressures can spur mental health conditions in new moms and dads.* Press Release. http://www.asanet.org/press/super_parent_cultural_pressures.cfm.

Bernard, K., Nissim, G., Vaccaro, S., Harris, J. L., & Lindhiem, O. (2018). Association between maternal depression and maternal sensitivity from birth to 12 months: A meta-analysis. *Attachment & Human Development, 20*(6), 578–599. https://doi.org/10.1080/14616734.2018.1430839.

Bryson, H., Perlen, S., Price, A., Mensah, F., Gold, L., Dakin, P., & Goldfeld, S. (2021). Patterns of maternal depression, anxiety, and stress symptoms from pregnancy to 5 years postpartum in an Australian cohort experiencing adversity. *Archives of Women's Mental Health, 24*(6), 987–997. https://doi.org/10.1007/s00737-021-01145-0.

Centre of Perinatal Excellence (COPE). (2017). Mental health care in the perinatal period: Australian clinical practice guideline. https://cdn.sanity.io/files/2eln2asx/production/bcb60218b0fcb81fb0dc0b516e4e1ef69b4ae4d6.pdf

Dayan, J., Creveuil, C., Marks, M. N., Conroy, S., Herlicoviez, M., Dreyfus, M., & Tordjman, S. (2006). Prenatal depression, prenatal anxiety, and spontaneous preterm birth: A prospective cohort study among women with early and regular care. *Psychosomatic Medicine, 68*(6), 938–946. https://doi.org/10.1097/01.psy.0000244025.20549.bd.

Dennis, C. L., Falah-Hassani, K., & Shiri, R. (2017). Prevalence of antenatal and postnatal anxiety: Systematic review and meta-analysis. *The British Journal of Psychiatry, 210*(5), 315–323. https://doi.org/10.1192/bjp.bp.116.187179.

Falah-Hassani, K., Shiri, R., & Dennis, C. L. (2017). The prevalence of antenatal and postnatal co-morbid anxiety and depression: a meta-analysis. *Psychological Medicine, 47*(12), 2041–2053. https://doi.org/10.1017/S0033291717000617.

Leach, L. S., Poyser, C., & Fairweather-Schmidt, K. (2017). Maternal perinatal anxiety: A review of prevalence and correlates. *Clinical Psychologist, 21*(1), 4–19. doi: 10.1111/cp.12058

Marmorstein, N. R., Malone, S. M., & Iacono, W. G. (2004). Psychiatric disorders among offspring of depressed mothers: Associations with paternal psychopathology. *American Journal of Psychiatry, 161*(9), 1588–1594. https://doi.org/10.1176/appi.ajp.161.9.1588.

Milgrom, J., Westley, D., & Gemmill, A. W. (2004). The mediating role of maternal responsiveness in some longer term effects of postnatal depression on infant development. *Infant Behaviour and Development, 27*(4), 443–454. https://doi.org/10.1016/j.infbeh.2004.03.003.

Rahman, A., Surkan, P. J., Cayetano, C. E., Rwagatare, P., & Dickson, K. E. (2013). Grand challenges: integrating maternal mental health into maternal and child health programmes. *PLoS medicine, 10*(5), e1001442.

Therapeutic Goods Administration. (2011). *Australian categorisation system for prescribing medicines in pregnancy.* Department of Health, Australian Government, 4 May 2011. https://www.tga.gov.au/australian-categorisation-system-prescribing-medicines-pregnancy.

VanderKruik, R., Barreix, M., Chou, D., Allen, T., Say, L., & Cohen, L. S. (2017). The global prevalence of postpartum psychosis: A systematic review. *BMC Psychiatry, 17*(1), 1–9. https://doi.org/10.1186/s12888-017-1427-7.

Wormser, H., Rieger, M., Domogalla, C., Kahnt, A., Buchwald, J., Kowatsch, M., Kuehnert, N., Buske-Kirschbaum, A., Papousek, M., Pirke, K.-M., & von Voss, H. (2006). Association between life stress during pregnancy and infant crying in the first six months postpartum: A prospective longitudinal study. *Early Human Development, 82*(5), 341–349. https://doi.org/10.1016/j.earlhumdev.2005.09.016.

FURTHER READING

Pairman, S., Tracy, S. K., Dahlen, H., & Dixon, S. (2022). *Midwifery: Preparation for Practice* (5th ed.). Elsevier.

Chapter 14

Chappell, L. C., Cluver, C. A., Kingdom, J., & Tong, S. (2021). Pre-eclampsia. *The Lancet, 398*(10297), 341–354. https://doi.org/10.1016/S0140-6736(20)32335-7.

Gestational Hypertension and Preeclampsia: ACOG Practice Bulletin, Number 222. (2020). *Obstetrics and Gynecology, 135*(6), e237–e260. https://doi.org/10.1097/AOG.0000000000003891.

Lowe, S. A., Bowyer, L., Lust, K., McMahon, M., North, R. A., Paech, M., Said, J. M. (2014). *Guideline for the Management of Hypertensive Disorders of Pregnancy.* https://ranzcog.edu.au/wp-content/uploads/2022/05/Guideline-for-the-Management-of-Hypertensive-Disorders-of-Pregnancy.pdf

Pairman, S., Tracy, S. K., Dahlen, H., & Dixon, S. (2022). *Midwifery: Preparation for Practice* (5th ed.). Elsevier.

Sakurai, S., Shishido, E., & Horiuchi, S. (2022). Experiences of women with hypertensive disorders of pregnancy: A scoping review. *BMC Pregnancy and Childbirth, 22*(1), 146. https://doi.org/10.1186/s12884-022-04463-y.

Serlachius, A., Hames, J., Juth, V., Garton, D., Rowley, S., & Petrie, K. J. (2018). Parental experiences of family-centred care from admission to discharge in the neonatal intensive care unit. *Journal of Paediatrics and Child Health, 54*(11), 1227–1233. https://doi.org/10.1111/jpc.14063.

World Health Organization (WHO). (2018). *Preterm birth.* https://www.who.int/news-room/fact-sheets/detail/preterm-birth

Chapter 15

Australian College of Midwives. (2021). *National midwifery guidelines for consultation and referral* (4th ed.). ACM. https://midwives.org.au/common/Uploaded%20files/_ADMIN-ACM/National-Midwifery-Guidelines-for-Consultation-and-Referral-4th-Edition-(2021).pdf.

Hanson, K. (2022). Why some parents dislike the term 'rainbow baby'. Today. https://www.today.com/parents/rainbow-baby-why-some-parents-dislike-term-t233195

Ho, A. L., Hernandez, A., Robb, J. M., Zeszutek, S., Luong, S., Okada, E., & Kumar, K (2022). Spontaneous miscarriage management experience: A systematic review. *Cureus, 14*(4), e24269. https://doi.org/10.7759/cureus.24269.

Jones, K., Robb, M., Murphy, S., & Davies, A. (2019). New understandings of fathers' experiences of grief and loss following stillbirth and neonatal death: A scoping review. *Midwifery, 79*, Article 102531. https://doi.org/10.1016/j.midw.2019.102531.

Lee, G. (2022). P6 – An audit of the Early Pregnancy Assessment Service: A retrospective cohort study. *Women and Birth, 35*(S1), 43–44. https://doi.org/10.1016/j.wombi.2022.07.121.

Meaney, S., Everard, C. M., Gallagher, S., & O'Donoghue, K (2017). Parents' concerns about future pregnancy after stillbirth: A qualitative study. *Health Expectations, 20*(4), 555–562. https://doi.org/10.1111/hex.12480.

Nursing and Midwifery Board of Australia (NMBA). (2018). *Midwife standards for practice.* https://www.nursingmidwiferyboard.gov.au/Codes-Guidelines-Statements/Professional-standards/Midwife-standards-for-practice.aspx

Pairman, S., Tracy, S. K., Dahlen, H., & Dixon, S. (2022). *Midwifery: Preparation for Practice* (5th ed.). Elsevier.

Pinnaduwage, L., Honeyford, J., Lackie, E., & Tunde-Byass, M. (2018). The sustained value of an Early Pregnancy Assessment Clinic in the management of early pregnancy complications: A 10-year retrospective study. *Journal of Obstetrics and Gynaecology Canada, 40*(8), 1017–1023. https://doi.org/10.1016/j.jogc.2017.12.002.

Rumbold, A. R., Yelland, J., Stuart-Butler, D., Forbes, M., Due, C., Boyle, F. M., & Middleton, P. (2020). Addressing stillbirth inequities in Australia: Steps towards a better future. *Women and Birth, 33*(6), 520–525. https://doi.org/10.1016/j.wombi.2020.08.012.

FURTHER READING

Stillbirth Foundation Australia. (2022). Pregnancy after loss. https://stillbirthfoundation.org.au/help-and-support/pregnancy-after-loss/

WEBSITES

Stillbirth and Newborn Death Support: https://www.sands.org.au/

Stillbirth Foundation Australia: https://stillbirthfoundation.org.au/

Chapter 16

Newman, J. E., Paul, R. C., & Chambers, G. M. (2021). *Assisted reproductive technology in Australia and New Zealand 2019.* Sydney: National Perinatal Epidemiology and Statistics Unit, the University of New South Wales.

Wang, R., Danhof, N. A., Tjon-Kon-Fat, R. I., Eijkemans, M. J. C., Bossuyt, P. M. M., Mochtar, M. H., van der Veen, F., Bhattacharya, S., Mol, B. J., & van Wely, M. (2019). Interventions for unexplained infertility: A systematic review and meta-analysis. *Cochrane Database of Systematic Reviews, 9*, Article CD012692. Art. No.:. https://doi.org/10.1002/14651858.CD012692.pub2.

FURTHER READING

Pairman, S., Tracy, S. K., Dahlen, H., & Dixon, S. (2022). *Midwifery: Preparation for Practice* (5th ed.). Elsevier.

Chapter 17

Australian College of Midwives. (2021), *National midwifery guidelines for consultation and referral* (4th ed.). https://midwives.org.au/common/Uploaded%20files/_ADMIN-ACM/National-Midwifery-Guidelines-for-Consultation-and-Referral-4th-Edition-(2021).pdf.

Australian Commission on Safety and Quality in Health Care (ACSQHC). (2021). *High rates of early caesarean sections are putting Australian babies at unnecessary risk.* https://www.safetyandquality.gov.au/about-us/latest-news/media-releases/high-rates-early-caesarean-sections-are-putting-australian-babies-unnecessary-risk

Australian Institute of Health and Welfare (AIHW). (2022). *National core maternity indicators: Caesarean section.* Australian Government. https://www.aihw.gov.au/reports/mothers-babies/national-core-maternity-indicators-1/contents/labour-and-birth-indicators/caesarean-section.

Betrán, A. P., Temmerman, M., Kingdon, C., Mohiddin, A., Opiyu, N., Torlini, M. R., Zhang, J., Musana, O., Wanyonyi, S. Z., Gülmezoglu, A. M., & Downe, S. (2018). Interventions to reduce unnecessary caesarean sections in healthy women and babies. *The Lancet, 392*(10155), 1358–1368. https://doi.org/10.1016/S0140-6736(18)31927-5.

Dahlen, H. G., Tracy, S., Tracy, M., Bisits, A., Brown, C., & Thornton, C. (2014). Rates of obstetric intervention and associated perinatal mortality and morbidity among low-risk women giving birth in public and private hospitals in NSW (2000–2008): A linked data population-based cohort study. *BMJ Open, 4*(5), Article e004551. https://doi.org/10.1136/bmjopen-2013-004551.

Davis, D., Homer, C. S., Clack, D., Turkmani, S., & Foureur, M. (2020). Choosing vaginal birth after caesarean section: Motivating factors. *Midwifery, 88*, 1–6. https://doi.org/10.1016/j.midw.2020.102766.

Devarajan, S., Talaulikar, V. S., & Arulkumaran, S. (2018). Vaginal birth after caesarean. *Obstetrics, Gynaecology & Reproductive Medicine, 28*(4), 110–115. https://doi.org/10.1016/j.ogrm.2018.02.001.

Finucane, E. M., Murphy, D. J., Biesty, L. M., Gyte, G. L. M., Cotter, A. M., Ryan, E. M, Boulvain, M., & Devane, D. (2020). Membrane sweeping for induction of labour. *Cochrane Datacase of Systematic Reviews, 2.* https://doi.org/10.1002/14651858.CD000451.pub3.

Fobelets, M., Beeckman, K., Faron, G., Daly, D., Begley, C., & Putman, K. (2018). Vaginal birth after caesarean versus elective repeat caesarean delivery after one previous caesarean section: A cost-effectiveness analysis in four European countries. *BMC Pregnancy and Childbirth, 18*(92), 1–10. https://doi.org/10.1186/s12884-018-1720-6.

Miller, Y. D., Tone, J., Talukdar, S., & Martin, E. (2022). A direct comparison of patient-reported outcomes and experiences in alternative models of maternity care in Queensland, Australia. *PLoS One, 17*(7), Article e0271105. https://doi.org/10.1371/journal.pone.0271105.

Pairman, S., Tracy, S. K., Dahlen, H., & Dixon, S. (2022). *Midwifery: Preparation for Practice* (5th ed.). Elsevier.

The Royal Hospital for Women. (2022). *Next birth after caesarean section (NBAC). Local operating procedure: Clinical policies, procedures and guidelines*. South Eastern Sydney Local Health District. https://www.seslhd.health.nsw.gov.au/sites/default/files/documents/Next_Birth_After_Caesarean_Section_1.pdf.

Chapter 18

Bovbjerg, M., Cheyney, M., & Caughey, A. (2021). Maternal and neonatal outcomes following waterbirth: A cohort study of 17 530 waterbirths and 17 530 propensity score-matched land births. *BJOG: an International Journal of Obstetrics and Gynaecology, 129*(6), 950–958. https://doi.org/10.1111/1471-0528.17009.

Clews, C., Church, S., & Ekberg, M. (2020). Women and waterbirth: A systematic meta-synthesis of qualitative studies. *Women and Birth: Journal of the Australian College of Midwives, 33*(6), 566–573. https://doi.org/10.1016/j.wombi.2019.11.007.

Cluett, E. R., Burns, E., & Cuthbert, A. (2018). Immersion in water during labour and birth. *Cochrane Database of Systematic Reviews, 5*(5), Article CD000111. https://doi.org/10.1002/14651858.CD000111.pub4.

Pairman, S., Tracy, S. K., Dahlen, H., & Dixon, S. (2022). *Midwifery: Preparation for Practice* (5th ed.). Elsevier.

Ulfsdottir, H., Saltvedt, S., Ekborn, M., & Georgsson, S. (2018). Like an empowering micro-home: A qualitative study of women's experience of giving birth in water. *Midwifery, 67*, 26–31. https://doi.org/10.1016/j.midw.2018.09.004.

Chapter 19

Dahlen, H., Jackson, M., Schmied, V., Tracy, S., & Priddis, H. (2011). Birth centres and the national maternity services review: Response to consumer demand or compromise? *Women and Birth: Journal of the Australian College of Midwives, 24*(4), 165–172. https://doi.org/10.1016/j.wombi.2010.11.001.

Davis, D. L., & Homer, C. S. E. (2016). Birthplace as the midwife's work place: How does place of birth impact on midwives? *Women and Birth, 29*(5), 407–415. https://doi.org/10.1016/j.wombi.2016.02.004.

Forster, D. A., McLachlan, H. L., Davey, M. A., Biro, M. A., Farrell, T., Gold, L., Flood, M., Shafiei, T., & Waldenström, U. (2016). Continuity of care by a primary midwife (caseload midwifery) increases women's satisfaction with antenatal, intrapartum and postpartum care: Results from the COSMOS randomised controlled trial. *BMC Pregnancy and Childbirth, 16*, 28. https://doi.org/10.1186/s12884-016-0798-y.

Homer, C., Brodie, P., & Leap, N. (2019). *Midwifery continuity of care*. Churchill-Livingstone Australia.

Homer, C. S. E., Cheah, S. L., Rossiter, C., Dahlen, H. G., Ellwood, D., Foureur, M. J., Forster, D. A., McLachlan, H. L., Oats, J. J. N., Sibbritt, D., Thornton, C., & Scarf, V. L. (2019). Maternal and perinatal outcomes by planned place of birth in Australia 2000–2012: A linked population data study. *BMJ Open, 9*(10). https://doi.org/10.1136/bmjopen-2019-029192.

Nursing and Midwifery Board of Australia. (2022). *Endorsement for scheduled medicines for midwives*. file:///C:/Users/amc302/Dropbox/PC/Downloads/Fact-sheet-Nursing-and-Midwifery-Board—Fact-sheet—Endorsement-for-scheduled-medicines-for-midwives%20(1).PDF

Sandall, J., Soltani, H., Gates, S., Shennan, A., & Devane, D. (2016). Midwife-led continuity models versus other models of care for childbearing women. *Cochrane Database of Systematic Reviews, 4*. https://doi.org/10.1002/14651858.CD004667.pub5.

Sidery, S. (2014). *Sheryl Sidery: Authentic, intuitive, sensitive midwifery.* http://www.sherylsidery.com

FURTHER READING

Pairman, S., Tracy, S. K., Dahlen, H., & Dixon, S. (2022). *Midwifery: Preparation for Practice* (5th ed.). Elsevier.

Chapter 20

Australian Institute of Health and Welfare (AIHW). (2022). *Congenital anomalies in Australia*. Australian Government. https://www.aihw.gov.au/reports/mothers-babies/congenital-anomalies-in-australia-2016/contents/congenital-anomalies-in-australia.

Moore, K. L., Persaud, T. V. N., & Torchia, M. G. (2016). *Before we are born: Essentials of embryology and birth defects* (9th ed.). Elsevier.

World Health Organization (WHO). (2023). *Congenital disorders*. https://www.who.int/health-topics/congenital-anomalies#tab=tab_1

FURTHER READING

Pairman, S., Tracy, S. K., Dahlen, H., & Dixon, S. (2022). *Midwifery: Preparation for Practice* (5th ed.). Elsevier.

Chapter 21

Australian Bureau of Statistics (ABS). (2022). *Cultural diversity of Australia*. https://www.abs.gov.au/articles/cultural-diversity-australia

Australian Human Rights Commission (AHRC). (2014). *Face the facts: Cultural diversity*. https://www.abs.gov.au/articles/cultural-diversity-australia

Australian Institute of Health and Welfare. (2019). *Towards estimating the prevalence of female genital mutilation/cutting in Australia*. Australian Government. https://www.aihw.gov.au/getmedia/f210a1d8-5a3a-4336-80c5-ca6bdc2906d5/aihw-phe-230.pdf.aspx?inline=true.

Australian Institute of Health and Welfare. (2022). *Australia's mothers and babies: Maternal country of birth*. Australian Government. https://www.aihw.gov.au/reports/mothers-babies/australias-mothers-babies/contents/demographics-of-mothers-and-babies/maternal-country-of-birth.

Department of Health and Aged Care. (2020). *Pregnancy care guidelines: Pregnancy care for migrant and refugee women*. https://www.health.gov.au/resources/pregnancy-care-guidelines/part-a-optimising-pregnancy-care/pregnancy-care-for-migrant-and-refugee-women

Hogan, R., Rossiter, C., & Catling, C. (2018). Cultural empathy in midwifery students: Assessment of an education program. *Nurse Education Today, 70*, 103–108. https://doi.org/10.1016/j.nedt.2018.08.023.

Miller, S., & Bear, R. J. (2022). Midwifery partnership. In S. Pairman, S. K. Tracy, H. Dahlen, & L. Dixon (Eds.), *Midwifery preparation for practice* (5th ed., pp. 355–392). Elsevier.

Multicultural Health Communication Service (MHCS). (2022). *Resource search: Maternal health*. https://www.mhcs.health.nsw.gov.au/publications/resource-search/?collectionfilter=1&fc_check=4a7035d4bc2e8eea eac8db127efcf4bf&fc_ends=120&Subject=Maternal+Health

Nursing and Midwifery Board of Australia (NMBA). (2018). *Midwife standards for practice*. https://www.nursingmidwiferyboard.gov.au/Codes-Guidelines-Statements/Professional-standards/Midwife-standards-for-practice.aspx

WEBSITES

The World Health Organization website provides information on female genital mutilation. Available at: http://www.who.int/topics/female_genital_mutilation/en/http://www.who.int/mediacentre/factsheets/fs241/en/

Female Genital Mutilation (FGM) in New Zealand: https://fgm.co.nz/

Australian Government Review of Australia's FGM legal framework: https://nla.gov.au/nla.obj-2817044791/view

FURTHER READING

Billett, H., Vazquez Corona, M., & Bohren, M. A. (2022). Women from migrant and refugee backgrounds' perceptions and experiences of the continuum of maternity care in Australia: A qualitative evidence synthesis. *Women and Birth, 35*(4), 327–339. https://doi.org/10.1016/j.wombi.2021.08.005.

Momoh, C. (Ed.). (2005). *Female genital mutilation.* Radcliffe Publishing.

Pairman, S., Tracy, S. K., Dahlen, H., & Dixon, S. (2022). *Midwifery: Preparation for Practice* (5th ed.). Elsevier.

Pregnancy, Birth and Baby. (2021). *Cultural practices and preferences when having a baby.* https://www.pregnancybirthbaby.org.au/cultural-practices-and-preferences-when-having-a-baby

RCOG Statement No. 53, May 2009. *Female Genital Mutilation and its management.* https://www.rcog.org.uk/globalassets/documents/guidelines/gtg-53-fgm.pdf

Royal Women's Hospital, The. (2020). *Female genital mutilation/cutting – Guideline for care.* https://thewomens.r.worldssl.net/images/uploads/downloadable-records/clinical-guidelines/female-genital-mutilation-cutting-guideline-for-care_280720.pdf

Simpson, J., Robinson, K., Creighton, S., & Hodes, D. (2012). Female Genital Mutilation: The role of health professionals in prevention, assessment and management. *BMJ, 344,* e542.

Turkmani, S., Homer, C., & Dawson, A. (2018). Maternity care experiences and health needs of migrant women from female genital mutilation–practicing countries in high-income contexts: A systematic review and meta-synthesis. *Birth, 46*(1), 3–14. http://dx.doi.org/10.1111/birt.12367.

Turkmani, S., Homer, C., Varol, N., & Dawson, A. (2018). A survey of Australian midwives' knowledge, experience, and training needs in relation to female genital mutilation. *Women and Birth, 31*(1), 25–30.

Chapter 22

Benzie, C., Newton, M., Forster, D., & McLachlan, H. (2022). How are women with a disability identified in maternity services in Australia? A cross-sectional survey of maternity managers. *Women and Birth, 36*(1), e161–e168. https://doi.org/10.1016/j.wombi.2022.06.002.

Malouf, R., Henderson, J., & Redshaw, M. (2017). Access and quality of maternity care for disabled women during pregnancy, birth and the postnatal period in England: Data from a national survey. *BMJ Open, 7*(7), Article e016757. https://doi.org/10.1136/bmjopen-2017-016757.

Nursing and Midwifery Board of Australia (NMBA). (2018). *Midwife standards for practice.* https://www.nursingmidwiferyboard.gov.au/Codes-Guidelines-Statements/Professional-standards/Midwife-standards-for-practice.aspx

Pituch, E., Bindiu, A. M., Grondin, M., & Bottari, C. (2022). Parenting with a physical disability and cognitive impairments: A scoping review of the needs expressed by parents. *Disability & Rehabilitation, 44*(13), 3285–3300. https://doi.org/10.1080/09638288.2020.1851786.

Smithson, C. A., McLachlan, H. L., Newton, M. S., Smith, C., & Forster, D. A. (2021). Perinatal outcomes of women with a disability who received pregnancy care through a specialised disability clinic in Melbourne, Australia. *Australian & New Zealand Journal of Obstetrics & Gynaecology, 61*(4), 548–553. https://doi.org/10.1111/ajo.13326.

Williams, N. (2021). Working with women who have a disability. *Australian Midwifery News, 25*(1), 44–45. https://search.informit.org/doi/abs/10.3316/informit.984044496248849.

WEBSITES

Women with individual needs clinic at the Royal Women's Hospital (Melbourne): https://www.thewomens.org.au/health-professionals/maternity/women-with-individual-needs

disAbility Maternity Care, a community-based organisation committed to supporting and empowering parents with disabilities, providing resources and training: https://www.disabilitymaternitycare.com/

The WashHouse, a community-based resource centre that aims to reduce violence and social disadvantage for women and girls: https://www.washhouse.org.au/

FURTHER READING

Pairman, S., Tracy, S. K., Dahlen, H., & Dixon, S. (2022). *Midwifery: Preparation for Practice* (5th ed.). Elsevier.

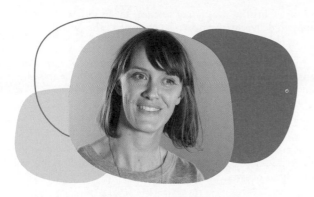

CHAPTER 1

Sarah's story

My name's Sarah and this is Isla. And I had my baby with the midwifery group practice at a public hospital in Sydney.

My pregnancy was easy, as far as pregnancies go. I didn't have any nausea or any complications. I felt really good the whole time and I gave birth at 3 days before my due day. As part of the group practice, I just had regular appointments, generally with the same midwife. Which was great. It meant I did know who I was seeing every week, and I always felt confident that we were on the same wavelength and that they understood who I was and what I was going through. And I also had a student midwife who was with me the whole time.

In the group practice, there were a number of midwives. I usually saw one, Christine, every visit. There were a few times I met other midwives which was encouraged because you don't know who's going to be on shift on the day you give birth. So in the end, I probably met about four of the other midwives. All of them were lovely, I felt really comfortable with them. And I just happened to be lucky that I got my midwife on the day. She happened to be on shift when I went into labour.

I feel like I had a really good relationship with Christine, my midwife. I feel like we were on the same page, we had a similar sort of sense of humour. I quite enjoyed seeing her every appointment. It wasn't like a doctor's appointment, it was sort of meeting up with someone for a chat. And you happened to be also having … she was also checking my measurements, checking I was okay. It was very casual and that was really nice. Most visits Tammy, the student, would come as well, and sometimes she would actually run the appointment, just to get more experience. And I always felt really comfortable with both of them. It was something I didn't feel with the GP I'd seen at the beginning. I felt really disheartened at the beginning and so when I did get into this group practice, it was such a relief. I can't explain how relieved I was to be able to have my pregnancy and birth the way I really had always envisioned it. So I feel incredibly fortunate to be able to have that opportunity.

My birth experience

So my birth experience was quite straightforward. I was lucky in that I spent most of it at home. I laboured for about 11 hours before, at the urging of my husband, to finally go to the hospital. We rang the midwife a couple of times and I seemed to be managing the pain quite well so I don't think they thought I needed to come in as urgently as my husband did. And we got there with an hour to spare, just enough time to fill the bath. And she arrived very suddenly, shot out. She had the cord around her neck a couple of times, but she was fine. She came out, got her colour really quickly and had a very healthy set of lungs when she emerged. And everything was okay.

To manage the contractions, I did a lot of breathing and a lot of sound, which … I'd take big breaths in and sort of made a lot of sound as the end of the wave, I suppose. I found that made a huge difference. I think it was something else to concentrate on, rather than the contractions.

My husband helped me through the labour by being in the room at all times. I remember him saying to me, just go back to sleep, we were told we should rest. And I thought, 'That's not going to happen and you're going to be with me the whole time'. And it progressed quite quickly and I just wanted him to be with me the whole time. I didn't expect him to do anything; I knew there's not much he can do. But I just felt a lot more comfortable and felt I could get through each contraction if he was there to hold my hand.

Having a water birth was something that I was really hoping I could do when I was thinking about having a baby. I thought I'd also need the shower more when I was at home, but it turns out that was incredibly uncomfortable. It wasn't something that actually made me feel any better. But as soon as I got in the bath at the hospital, everything just slowed down a little bit. I felt a bit more in control. Just the adrenaline sort of calmed down a bit and I just felt calmer.

And she shot out really quickly. And I just remember sort of bringing her to the surface and just sort of watching all the colours change on her skin. And looking at her, I just couldn't believe how alert she was, like, just there were these big eyes and she looked like a person. That was really … I don't know why that surprised me but it was this abstract thing that was now real.

So I was actually really glad when I rang and knew that at 7 am, Christine was going to come on to shift and I could hopefully deliver when she was there. I would have been happy to deliver with any of the midwives. That was the good thing about the group practice. I knew almost all of them or at least met them once.

But there was something nice about being able to share that with her because she's the person I'd seen the most. And it was also really nice to have the student midwife there, for her to arrive at the last minute. And just have the only people in the room were the student and the midwife and my husband. So it was really intimate. It didn't feel intrusive; it was just exactly what I wanted for my birth.

I think we had 4 hours in the room to ourselves in the birth centre.

We sat in the double bed and we just had a chance to just be, we were just left to our own devices. And that was not intrusive. We didn't have any visitors, it was just a chance to get to know each other. And once she stopped crying, we could finally realise what had happened. We were now three instead of two.

Breastfeeding

I attempted breastfeeding pretty much straight away. She definitely had a good suck; she just wasn't sucking on the right part. She wasn't quite latching on, but she definitely knew what she was doing. So I wasn't really worried about it. But it was nice, like straight away, having that help. It was something that obviously is very important at the beginning. And so straight away the student midwife was helping me trying to latch on and she was very encouraging.

I think by the end of the first week we were more than established. I think I was really lucky, my husband was very helpful. I think he couldn't believe how hard breastfeeding actually could be at the beginning. I mean there were definitely tears, as you get quite stressed 'cause all you're thinking is, 'I just want to feed my baby, and she's hungry'. And it takes a few days, obviously, for the milk to come in. And you've got hormones and it feels very overwhelming at first. But once it's established, it was like, it just feels like such a good achievement.

Like you have this relationship that's, I don't know how to describe it really. It's just like I could give her something, like more than just holding her. Like I could feed her, I was giving her life.

Midwifery support with early mothering

The first few days I stayed two nights in the hospital. I'm glad I did that, I think. I could have gone home probably earlier. I was more than … I recovered really well; it was a very straightforward birth. But I'm just glad I had the midwives on call when I had any questions. Especially with the breastfeeding, I just really wanted to leave the hospital feeling confident that I was doing the right thing. And just having that buzzer in the middle of the night—saying, 'Why is she doing this?' or 'Why won't she settle?'—that was very comforting. I'm very glad I didn't go home straight away.

I remember feeling really glad that when we arrived home that we would have a midwife visit the next day. So we arrived home on the Saturday and a midwife gave us a call. And she came and visited us on the Sunday. And we had another visit about 4 days later. So the first visit was when every member of our family was also over. That felt a bit crazy. She told us we're doing okay, what we should watch out for, just reminding us to wake her up to feed her and helping a little bit more with the breastfeeding, which still was a bit touch and go. And by the time we had the next visit, about 4 days later, she was attaching a lot better. We really only needed those two visits. I did get another phone call later to ask if we wanted another visit. But we were feeling pretty good. We figured it was okay, we could go forward without any more help.

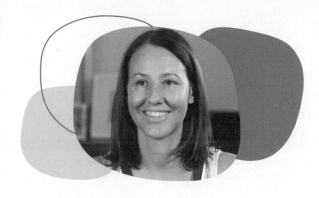

CHAPTER 1

Tamara

My name's Tamara Ellis. I've recently completed my 3-year Bachelor of Midwifery. I'm currently working as a new graduate midwife. I have been for a few months now.

Continuity of care experiences

As a midwifery student, I completed 35 continuity of care experiences. The course requirement was 30 and I did extra. I really enjoyed doing them.

Continuity of care helped my learning as a midwifery student in many different ways. Firstly, as a student, we worked in the GP shared care system at the hospital. My hospital actually had two models of care: GP shared care and the group practice caseload midwives. And generally as a student, we worked in the GP shared care system. In third year we did a brief stint with the continuity of care MGP midwives.

So the continuity of care experiences enabled me to work with women throughout the whole continuum of pregnancy, through their antenatal experiences, their labour experiences, their birth experiences and their early days as a mother. So it really did enable me to see birth's not just about that one day, turning up in the birthing unit, the woman having her baby, catching her baby; it's so much more than that. It's about the whole journey, the pregnancy journey, the journey of becoming a mother. And I guess working with a woman and a family throughout that whole experience for a woman, really enables you to see that.

Another thing I learnt, I guess, is I always felt much more comfortable practising my midwifery skills with a woman that I knew and that I'd developed a relationship with. And they were all also generally quite keen to help your learning as well. They really enjoyed … it's such a reciprocal relationship, I found. You supported them and answered questions and helped them and they mostly really enjoyed the fact that they were helping your learning.

It also gave me a lot of opportunities. I tried to make the most of that. A lot of opportunities to increase my learning. Whether it be in the antenatal clinic, in the birthing unit or sometimes women would need to be referred on, they'd need to go to the pregnancy day stay unit, and making the most of those opportunities as well for extra learning. I found that really helpful.

We don't get a lot of clinical experience. So I saw continuity of care as an opportunity for me to just gain as much clinical experience as I could, and I really enjoyed that. And support her through that and be a familiar face through all of that, rather than somebody going through that generally fragmented hospital system and not knowing anyone and getting lost in that system. You were, as a student, often a constant for that woman through those experiences.

Setting professional boundaries

So I found … one of the things that I really found helpful in my learning was learning to set professional and personal boundaries with women. This is something in the beginning I found really difficult. So for me, over the course of 3 years, I found that very helpful and I can see how much I progressed in that way over the 3 years. And my 'continuity of care' women definitely helped me, helped me with that.

I also found that women often confided in me and I would … for example, I had one woman who had confided that she had a history of sexual abuse. So learning to keep trust, keep that trust going, but also realising that things like that were often out of my scope of practice, and how to deal with those situations. And we actually got her a place in one of the group practices with a group practice midwife. I worked with that midwife and with that woman throughout her pregnancy, again seeing the referrals that took place. And then being there at her birth and seeing how much of a difference that these things made to her and made to her birth and made to her experience. And then how much that affected her transition into motherhood as well.

I could really see how that continuity of care and that experience, in particular, helped her so much in having a normal birth. And in feeling safe and having a good experience and how important that was for her in healing, in a small way, and also in her transition to motherhood and becoming a mother. It really was very valuable for her. And also very satisfying for me, as a student and as a student midwife, to see what a difference that made for her and the small part that I may have played in that and supporting her through such a difficult and amazing time.

Building relationships

For me, one of the best and most positive things about the continuity of care experiences was the relationships I had the opportunity to develop with women and their families, getting to know them quite intimately. And it was such an honour to be in that position, to watch them go through pregnancy, learn about their hopes, their fears, what they wanted for their birth, what their ideals were. And to be able to help them and support them with those things, to arrive at the birthing unit when they were in labour and to see their faces. They were mostly happy to see a face that they knew. And to watch them have their baby and to support them through that. And to see a family together following that, to see them with their little … their baby.

And not even necessarily the experience that they wanted or that they saw themselves having—sometimes things happen that are beyond anyone's control. But even in those instances, women, trying your best to make sure that they feel in control and that they feel informed and that they know what's going on and, really I always tried to do that, to spend that time.

Often the midwife herself would be very busy with that woman's care. So something as a student we can do, is just be with the woman, be with her and talk to her and reassure her and, if you can, be honest with her. And as a student this was something I felt I could do more than the midwife, just be with the woman, and that was fantastic.

Challenges with providing continuity of care

There were a couple of challenges, I found, with the continuity of care experiences. Namely these were, I guess, being on call; sometimes that was difficult. It was also exciting sometimes as well, but sometimes it was difficult. Especially in the early days, I think, before I really learnt to set limits. And I think I got a lot better at that as time progressed, as time went on over the 3 years.

Another difficulty I faced, or I found, was fitting in the continuity of care experiences with my uni life and my home life and my hospital clinical work. But I also found this was a good learning experience as well because time management is such an important thing to learn and is such another big learning curve as a midwife and I think that really helped. It has really helped me with time management.

Providing continuity of care to Sarah

My experiences in providing care to Sarah were fantastic, actually. I really enjoyed helping, or supporting, Sarah through her pregnancy journey. And she taught me so much. Sarah really had a fantastic outlook. And she really throughout, from the beginning, she trusted her body. She believed, just believed in normal birth. That was just the way she saw pregnancy and birth and that was fantastic.

I really learnt from her that, 'the less you do, the more you give'. Which I found quite a tricky concept to grasp. I sort of felt with her that I should be doing more, I should be, you know, as a student often I busied myself, I wanted to be seen as competent. But with Sarah, I really learnt that; that especially during her birth … I was just there and she was giving birth. It was her that was doing it all. I didn't need to do anything. And she did it, she gave birth on her own really. She did it all herself. She really trusted her body and she did it. And I learnt a lot from that.

Another thing I learnt with Sarah was just some insight into the transition into motherhood and early days of being a mother, of becoming a mother, becoming a family. I think Sarah's little baby, right from the moment she came out, was quite unsettled. So that was very challenging for her. And also breastfeeding was a bit of a challenge. So again, seeing those things through her eyes, the way she dealt with that, the way they as a family dealt with that.

Babies are unsettled. Babies do do that, it is normal. Breastfeeding is hard for many women. It is a learned thing for women and babies. And understanding that and explaining that, trying to help explain that to Sarah. And also seeing that myself, that it is normal and sitting with that. And just being there to support women and to tell them that it is normal. And to help them and to give them tips. And also for me learning from the midwife I worked with as well. Learning how she dealt with that with Sarah. The information and the wisdom that she could impart. Her knowledge of those things I learnt.

Also, being a part of Sarah's experience was great because Sarah was with a group practice. Her pregnancy care and her birth was with a group practice midwife. So that was great for me as well, working with that midwife. And really getting to know that midwife as well. And the three of us developed a good, professional relationship. And that was great, it was great learning for me as well.

Future midwifery goals

One day I would love to work in continuity of care, soon I hope. That's my goal. I'm trying to gain as much experience as I can. I'm trying to increase my skills as a midwife. I'm putting myself out of my comfort zone and learning suturing and learning different things that I will need as a group practice midwife with that goal in mind. That's something I would love to do. I just feel like it would be the ultimate for me, working across the continuum of pregnancy, labour, birth and early motherhood using all my skills as a midwife.

And it's funny actually, the group practice midwife that I did work with, we get on very well. And when I became a new graduate midwife, she said to me, 'I'd love you to join this group in the future sometime when you've done your new grad year. We'd love you to join our group'. So that was a confidence booster for me and something I would definitely love to pursue in the future.

Another great thing I found about the continuity of care experiences was the glimpses I got of how it is to be a real midwife. Working, I guess, working so closely with a woman throughout her pregnancy and birth, answering questions, referring women on to other care, being a bridge between the midwife and the woman, being on call. All of these things, sort of, gave me glimpses into how it is to be a real midwife. More than any other thing, I think. More than clinical experiences or anything else. It really gave you those insights into what it is to be a midwife. And to be with a woman and a family.

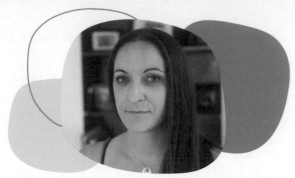

CHAPTER 1

Christine

I'm Christine Turner. I work in a publicly funded midwifery group practice model in a large tertiary hospital in Sydney.

Becoming a group practice midwife

I became a midwife providing continuity of care in midwifery group practice following my postgrad rotations. So I did a Bachelor of Midwifery and then I did a new grad rotation throughout all areas of the hospital. And a position became available once I'd finished my last placement and I wanted to make sure that I kept up all my skills. So in birthing, postnatally, antenatally. So I applied for it and got it and I've been working in it since then.

My degree focused a lot on continuity of care, which made me feel that that's what we were preparing ourselves for. We weren't preparing ourselves to be stuck in one place. So I feel it did prepare us to work in midwifery group practice.

The practical training we had was every aspect of midwifery and I was fortunate as a student to have a 2- or 3-month placement with a midwifery group practice at the hospital I'm currently working at, right at the end of my training. So it kind of brought everything together for me. So it just, was like a natural progression to go into midwifery group practice. Doing something else didn't actually make sense to me.

I chose to work this way because once I graduated I didn't want to be stuck working in one area. I wanted to use all the skills that I'd learnt. So I didn't want to be a midwife who became used to working just in postnatal or antenatal. I wanted to make sure that I continued using all the skills that I'd learnt.

The relationship with the women

The relationship with the women is one of the things that actually keeps me in the job. I've actually met some beautiful women who've come back for their second, third, even fourth babies with me. So for some of them I've known them for 5 years throughout their whole childbearing years. And I find you get feedback from the women that, when they come in, in labour and they know you, they don't feel like they need to tell you their story. They don't need to give you any information because you know them. And then following them up at home afterwards, once they've got their newborns, it's just nice to actually be able to go to into their environment; they feel relaxed.

Working with Sarah

When I was looking after Sarah throughout her pregnancy, she was absolutely lovely. I really enjoyed getting to know her throughout the pregnancy. Working in a group practice, I'm not always on call. So, you know, there was a chance that when she came in to labour I wouldn't have been on call. But I'm very glad that I was.

Sarah did remarkably well with her labour and birth. She did the majority of the labour at home. We ... our women call us when they're at home, so they call us for advice. So we obviously do a lot of education antenatally with women about things that you can use at home, tools to use at home. Things like massage, showers, heat packs, all of those sorts of things.

So we find a lot of our women feel very comfortable labouring for as long as they, you know, further along in their labour because they have had that education. And also they've got us on the phone. So we'll often speak to a woman two or three times before they actually come in. In Sarah's case, she actually came in and was fully dilated. So I guess that shows that she did feel confident and comfortable with labouring at home for that amount of time.

And we find that a lot of our women are like that. Not every woman, 'cause every woman's different. But a lot of our women do feel much more comfortable labouring as long as possible at home. And we find they ... less women come in too early or not in established labour. More women come in, you know, almost transitional or about to have a baby, which has been quite common with us lately.

And we just find that a lot of our women, they're not interested in pain relief options as much as, I suppose, the general population that you see in the hospital. So we have less rates of epidurals, less rates of intervention medically, less rate of caesarean section rate across the board with all of our women compared to the hospital, general population of women.

She had a really, really beautiful birth experience with myself and a student midwife who followed her through the whole experience as well. And then we did get to see her postnatally as well. And then again for her postnatal checks. So really for the whole process I was able to look after her. It was a joy to look after Sarah.

Having a student working with us in group practice

Having a student working with us in group practice is something that my group in particular really, really love. For us it's a great opportunity for us to teach and to show the students how we work.

Every midwife works slightly different and the feedback we get from students is that it's great to sort of see how different midwives do things. For them it's a … they can see how they want to work or how they may not want to work. So I think for them they find it very, very beneficial in that way, in an educational way.

And one student in particular that we had looking after one of our women following through was Tammy, who was following through Sarah. And I know that Sarah really enjoyed the relationship that she built with Tammy. Tammy was there for most of her appointments, she was there when she had her baby and I know that she saw her postnatally as well.

And I think that that relationship, on top of the relationship that I had with her, she had an extra person to feel comfortable with. And I think that that really had a big benefit for her and in how her pregnancy and labour and birth went. And I know that for the student it was very, very beneficial as well.

What the women say

One of the other things that women tell us is how intimate and private their birth experiences feel. So we try and maintain a calm environment, so unless we need someone for assistance it's generally just the midwife, sometimes the student midwife with the couple when they're having the baby. So a lot of women say it just felt nice and close and calm and quiet and intimate and private, which is what we hope to achieve and they're telling us that we're doing that so that's good.

Working in midwifery group practice

As the primary midwife, I provide care for four women per month. Within the group practice, being five midwives, so each of us having four women we're the primary carer for. So it equates to 20 women per month.

The best thing about working in this way for me, personally, is the professional relationships that I have. So working in a group with four other midwives, you're talking to each other on a daily basis. You have to communicate with each other about things. So you actually create really good friendships with them. And I think in any workplace, the people you work with make, you know, your life, your work enjoyable if you get along with them very, very well.

So that's one of the things that keeps me in the job—my workmates. And the other is because I'm not losing any skills. I've gained skills, you know, increasingly getting more skills. I just feel like I'm doing what a midwife should do. Doing the entire journey with the women.

I think one of the greatest challenges, working in my job, is things can get very hectic at times. So I may have a day where I have 10 appointments to see women antenatally. And then I get that phone call that I've got a woman in labour. So it can be a bit of a juggle trying to communicate with the women to say, 'We need to reschedule your appointment' while arranging when's the best time to get the woman in.

So there's a lot of juggling with time. You have to be really good at time management. You need to be able to realise how much time things are going to take so that you don't, you don't give yourself too short a time, or too much time for it. So it can be hectic juggling things around.

Some days are really, really busy, others are much quieter. And you find that, you know, you'll have a very busy week where every woman wants to have their baby in that week. And you just think please, just one day without a birth this week would be nice. But then you'll have a quiet week so it, it evens out. So sometimes you feel you're working long, long hours but then the next week you feel like you're not working that much at all.

I would definitely recommend midwives work in this way. I know it's not for everybody. I know that people have other things outside of work that, you know, they may not be able to work this way. But if you're wanting to maintain all your skills, all your midwifery skills, gain more skills, be autonomous—because you're very autonomous in this job, so I work out my day the way I need to. So anyone who wants to maintain skills, get along with people at work, be autonomous, I would definitely recommend it.

As well as working very closely within the group of midwives, we also have an obstetrician at the hospital who only looks after the women in our group specifically. We meet with her once a week so she knows if there's anything out of the ordinary, any complications arise, we refer to her. And she liaises very, very closely with us. The best thing about that is that even if something does happen with our women, we don't hand over care, we continue care. So we still, wherever their journey takes them, they've still got that continuity with the same group of midwives looking after them the whole way.

I think that continuity of care with women is actually really beneficial for helping women feel comfortable going home, establishing breastfeeding, getting used to what it's like to be a mother. So we try to establish breastfeeding as soon as the baby's born. So baby's put skin-to-skin on the mother's chest, and we assist women with establishing breastfeeding in the hospital so that they feel confident when they go home. So we go and see them for checks at home postnatally. It's very rare that I have a woman come back for her 6- to 8-week check-up and she's not breastfeeding. It's very rare.

CHAPTER 2

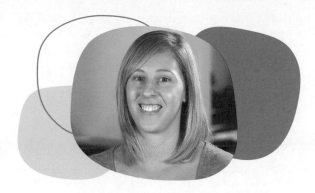

Kaitlin's story

I'm Kaitlin and I've just had a homebirth to Hunter, who is 8 weeks old now.

Deciding on having a homebirth

So Scott and I decided last year that we wanted to start our family. And so we went through a 4-month preconception period where we really cleaned up our diets, started taking a few supplements that we needed to ensure that we were, you know, as healthy as we possibly could be before we decided to try and fall pregnant. Which was great because we knew we would have clean, healthy bodies and then when it came time to start trying, it happened nearly straight away which was a really lovely relief for us. Also, I believe it really helped me through the pregnancy. 'Cause my pregnancy was very easy, I really didn't have any morning sickness, I was comfortable the whole time, so I enjoyed it. I really loved being pregnant. It was a great experience to feel Hunter growing inside me.

And when it came time for the birth, that was also a really wonderful experience as well. I was super-happy we chose homebirth because it just made me so comfortable in our surrounding, and the actual birth itself was lovely.

Once we were pregnant, we did start researching into what else was available: hospitals or birth centres. Mostly just using the internet and we'd talked to a few friends of ours as well. And through that we kind of found that a lot of people that we knew that had babies in hospital did have a lot of intervention and the birth never really went as planned, or was never as good as they were hoping for.

So because we were already predisposed to sort of wanting a homebirth and then having this information that we gathered about how safe homebirth was, and then how the hospital system was not exactly what we were looking for in this situation, that's when we decided, yes, we did want to have a homebirth and that's what we were very comfortable with.

So once we decided we were definitely having a homebirth, the next step was to start looking for a midwife. So we just Googled, really. We got onto a few different websites, found people who seemed to have a great reputation. And we'd organised a couple of interviews with different midwives—about three we had lined up—just to see how everyone differed, but Sheryl was actually the first one we interviewed. And once Scott and I left our meeting with her, we cancelled the other ones.

Preparing for birth

My pregnancy was very comfortable the whole way through. I tried to eat as healthily as possible and did plenty of yoga, kept up my exercise the whole way through. So even approaching the birth I found I still had quite a bit of energy which was great, very helpful. And I actually went a week overdue with Hunter, so we were very sure about our dates. I know that he was definitely one week over, but leading up to it was great. I didn't get particularly tired at all, which was nice. I was ready for him to come by that stage.

Sheryl was wonderful in talking to both of us about what our separate roles would be during the birth. So what I should be doing for myself to ensure that I was comfortable and getting everything that I needed and making sure that I could birth this baby as comfortably and safely as possible.

And then Scott's role as my support person to make sure he had everything ready and was listening to what I needed and observing all the different signs and making sure he knew what was going on as well. And when he should call her, and when he should not and we should just be by ourselves.

Labour and birth at home

When I actually woke up the morning that he was born, I still wasn't 100% sure that that's what was happening. I started to have a few sort of crampy feelings and I actually for some reason just thought it was cramps, not this could be the start of the birth. Even that, that was not painful. It was just, I felt like, I don't know, like I'd eaten something a bit off and was just having a few little cramps.

And then that was about 4 am, and I sort of went up and down to bed a couple of times. And then, after that … so that went on for a couple of hours. I tried to go back to sleep and back to bed, back to the bathroom. About 8 o'clock

Scott woke up and I said, 'Stay asleep, this is going to be a long haul'. We knew throughout all the pregnancy and the birth class we went to and talking with Sheryl as well, that we were in for sort of a 24-hour ride. So I wanted him to get as much sleep as possible.

However, about 9 o'clock, my water broke. So that was when I was like, 'Okay, probably time for you to get up now and start setting up things or at least getting ready for the day'. And from there […] progressed quite quickly. My contractions were coming, sort of a minute or two apart by 10 am, 10.30 am, which was fine because they weren't too intense.

That was, I guess, a saving grace of my homebirth. It was very comfortable the whole way through in terms of nothing got too intense, and when it did, it was over quite quickly. And Scott was a wonderful help in my birth, like he was the most amazing support partner there. He was the only person with me at that time for most of the birth. And so his help was just such a massive relief. He was doing some acupressure on my lower back which was just the most amazing pain relief I ever could have hoped for I think, during the birth, I never at one stage felt like I needed anything else. No medical pain relief, no drugs, nothing, because he was there doing that acupressure which was amazing.

His support there was just one of the biggest things that got me through the whole thing. I could not have done it without him there and guiding me and reminding me and just being there. Just being that loving support person who knew that everything was going to be okay. And reminding me of that the whole way through.

I felt like I probably wanted her to pop in and just check, and make sure everything was sort of progressing as it should be and was all going okay. I was a bit nervous and I think she had picked up by our phone calls that we were getting to that, sort of, nervous stage. And she wanted to come and just check on us and reassure us and make sure that everything was going okay and normal for us first timers who don't know all that much.

It's a steep learning curve, and as much as you hear about it and read about it and talk about it, it's very different to how it is on the day. So that when she arrived … sorry, so, we must have called her at 11 and she arrived by about 11.30. And yeah, was quite surprised to find that the baby was ready to come by then. So that was a nice surprise when she arrived, to hear that.

He was sort of right down low. She asked me to sort of feel, if I could feel his head. And it was only about a centimetre or less away from crowning, so that was quite intense to realise that it had all happened so quickly. So I had been labouring in the bathroom most of the time. I'd had a nice, hot shower, which really helped earlier in the labour with a bit of pain relief. And it was just really comfortable to be in there. So I'd been in there and then I was also using the support of the bathroom bench, just to lean on, while Scott helped me through each contraction.

So once she arrived and we realised that the baby was coming very, very soon, we moved out into the living room where the pool should have been set up.

So we created a nice little nest of towels and blankets just leaning over the coffee table, so in the middle of the living room floor. And the coffee table was nearby and we put a pillow on top of that. And so I gave birth to Hunter sort of on my knees leaning forward with my elbows on the coffee table. The actual birth itself, pushing him out, was wonderful. It was very intense. I wouldn't say painful.

Being in the upright position, I felt really helped a lot; it just felt natural and felt easy. And he came out beautifully. I think he got a little bit stuck with his head for one push. But Sheryl was there and she just said, 'No, no, stop pushing. Okay, start again and go'. And it was great, it was easy and he came out.

Sheryl had caught him on the way out and then just placed him on the floor between my legs on a towel. And so we just sort of … I was kneeling over him and we were just waiting for him to take his first breath. Which he did, a little gasp, which was amazing.

I think then I was just in a little bit of a trance, 'cause I, sort of, I was just staring at him. To the point where Sheryl was like, 'Okay, you should pick him up now'. So it must have only been about 10 seconds, but, yeah I picked him up. And then we wrapped him in a little blanket that we had ready to go. And then 'cause I was naked at that point as well, so I was wrapped up in a nice dressing gown, and we just moved straight up to the couch, which was wonderful being at home. I was just able to flop onto my own couch in my own dressing gown.

And we just sat there sort of cuddling and looking at, so then Scott joined us, just looking at our little boy which we discovered, at that point. Because we didn't know if we were having a boy or a girl. So that was wonderful. We just sat there for a few minutes looking at him going, 'Oh my gosh! Look at this amazing little person that's come out'.

So just after Hunter was born, we wrapped him up in a blanket and I was sort of wrapped up in a blanket and we were all cosy on the couch. And then we sort of sat and waited and looked for signs of him wanting the breast and wanting to feed. So I think that took, from memory, about 15 to 20 minutes.

And after that, so once we saw there were signs, Sheryl came over and really helped me to learn how to attach him properly. So she showed me how to get the nipple right into his mouth, make sure it's a deep attachment, that his mouth is fully over it and sucking it in, which was great 'cause he learnt that straight away which was really helpful to get that off the bat. So she stayed and watched him for, sort of, another hour or two.

Transition to parenthood

In Sheryl's visits when she came back every day, they were super-helpful. I was so glad to have her there. She helped with the breastfeeding, which was one thing that was obviously very important, but she also just told us about each of the daily, sort of, developmental steps that he would be taking.

I mean, I know they're not huge in those early days but it's amazing to just know that today they'll start, sort of, recognising your face and they'll start moving around. And more signs that he wants to feed. Obviously the first day it was just that little sucking motion, but as more signs came she would show us what they meant and how to deal with that. And then also just the practical things as well. Changing the nappies and how often they should be changed and cleaning him and making sure everything's nice and neat and dry and avoiding nappy rash and all those other little things that they can get.

And then also making sure that we understood that everything that was happening with him was normal because Hunter got quite a bad sort of rash of pimples all over his face and he looked like a 15-year-old boy. So to know that that was perfectly normal, a lot of babies did that, was great. You know, really reassuring as a first-time mum. And not having much experience with other little kids in my family, I really needed that support there to help me through.

I actually had a wonderful birth experience, so the days following that were really great for me.

Then as things went on … so second day was great, that day fortunately was quite quiet for us. I don't think we had many visitors. So Scott and Hunter and I were just all able to really spend a lot of time together and connect. Then Sheryl popping in was lovely and helping us through those daily needs that we had. The third day, sort of, once my milk came in, that was a crazy day, just having that new sensation was one thing and dealing with Hunter and he started to cry a little bit more by then.

I was quite overwhelmed, and that realisation that this is my life and this is forever, was a big deal for me. That happened around day 3 or 4. But, yeah, I was lucky in that I had the support of Sheryl and Scott and all of my family and Scott's family there.

So overall, my homebirth experience was absolutely wonderful. I couldn't recommend it more highly. Having Sheryl as my midwife was really an excellent support, because I met her so many times during the pregnancy. All our visits were very helpful, supportive. She taught me a lot of things about the technical side of birth, as well as the emotional support that she had there for me. And we really developed a lovely relationship, almost a friendship I would call it, throughout that time. And so having her then at the birth was even more special. And then having her come and visit each day after the birth and then the periodic visits after that. It's just … it's so lovely.

So the whole experience, I think was just absolutely wonderful and I have no doubt that for every other child I have after this, it'll be the same again. And hopefully with Sheryl again.

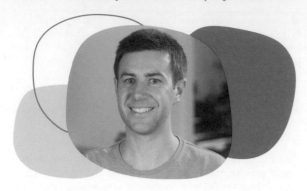

CHAPTER 2

Scott

My name is Scott. I'm Kaitlin's husband. And we had Hunter at home.

A father's decision to have a homebirth

My experience of the birth was a bit of a blur actually, now that I look back. It was fantastic overall, I guess I'd say. I have absolutely no regrets doing it at home. In fact, I'd rather, I actively try and tell my friends about the homebirth experience. Without trying to push it on them because that's more … first of all, if my mates don't have kids or aren't expecting kids, then, I don't want to talk about a birthing experience 'cause that's just a bit strange.

But if people ask me, I'm very happy to talk about it, 'cause that's something that we didn't really have. We had one friend that had a homebirth and that was it and so she was very happy to talk about it, but no one else.

And I think imparting our newfound wisdom, if you want to call it that, upon people is a good thing to do. Because even if it's just for education, I had no idea about what to expect with the birth really.

A father's experience of homebirth

The experience of the birth was very fast. Kait woke me up at 8 o'clock and said, 'I think something is happening'. That was pretty much all she said. At which point I started to go, 'Oh my god, it's on'. And then she said, 'But don't worry, I don't even know if it's real, I'm just getting a few pains. Go back to sleep, actually, I'll let you know'. And then so I did. Maybe that wasn't very responsible but she woke up at 9 o'clock and said, 'Something is happening, so get up'. And within 3 hours, he was born. So I had a half-eaten breakfast on the breakfast bar. Everything happened so fast.

She was, sort of, handling the contractions really well. In hindsight, she handled it amazingly well. It was almost like she was just riding it through, is the only way to describe it. She was just in the moment. She would talk to me in between contractions telling me what to do, say, 'Can I have another hot nappy, can I have a drink, can I have whatever, make me a smoothie', was one of the requests. I didn't get anywhere close to making the smoothie. But other than that, the contractions would come and she'd just be, sort of, in the moment.

I was applying some acupressure that we learnt at our birthing class. Which at the time, didn't feel like I was doing much at all. But post-birth, Kait told me it was the most amazing experience for her. It really made the pain subside and helped her out, which was great to know. But at the time, it felt like nothing to me. It's almost like, it's a bit surreal, I don't know how to explain it. It was like we were in a little bubble of our own world. Sort of, emotions were high and there was a real feeling in the air of something amazing, I guess.

I sort of felt like she was doing it all and I was just doing whatever I could to help her. That's sort of, that was my mindset. And then before we knew it, we had a baby, 'cause it came so quickly. When Sheryl came around, and she only made it by about 15 minutes, well that's what it felt like, the baby was out almost straight away. And I'm absolutely glad she was there to deliver it because I think I would have freaked out at that point in time.

But up until that point, everything felt completely in control. And that's probably because of Kait and all her research that she'd done and all her, both physical and mental preparation. She was completely in control and I was probably completely out of control. But trying to stay calm. That's how it felt to me.

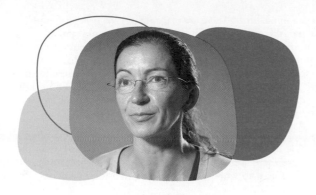

CHAPTER 3

Anke's story

I am Anke Reitter from Germany. I'm an obstetrician and I'm specialised in breech births and twin deliveries and I'm a maternal fetal medicine specialist. I started my training in UK in 1995 and basically I'm here in Australia for 6 months as a research fellow. And my main topic is the breech birth now.

My interest in vaginal breech birth started actually during my time in UK. During my training there were plenty of undiagnosed breech on labour ward. And that is how I got my training. And it happened in 1995 to 1999, so just before the Term Breech Trial. And that's why I had a very good opportunity to learn breech, yeah, as a young junior house officer and I loved it. And it was such a beautiful birth and I was so happy with a few manoeuvres I was able to help the baby out and I really enjoyed it. So that's why I was never fearful about breech vaginal birth.

Term Breech Trial

In terms of evidence base, the Term Breech Trial has been published in 2000 in *The Lancet* by a Canadian group. It was a multicentre trial and the main author was Hannah, from Canada. And basically since that time, overnight, the impact of this study was really, really there and overnight units have stopped offering vaginal breech births.

So all over the world there were people criticising the study and the conclusion of the study. And 2 years after the Term Breech Trial has been published, no sorry, 4 years, another study was published with follow-up data. And in this follow-up data, there was no difference between vaginal breech delivery and the planned caesarean group in term breech babies. So, but the study had already such an impact that units all over the world stopped overnight offering vaginal breech births. So that is the Term Breech Trial.

Training courses on vaginal breech birth

Yes, obstetrician who are keen on offering vaginal breech delivery often don't have a lot of experience themselves. But they want to offer the option. To be safe in offering the option of vaginal breech delivery, they could attend training courses and there are training courses for breech delivery, to be more confident in offering manoeuvres to help the baby if the arms are extended or if the head is not in an ideal position. And that can be trained very well with training models. And that has been studied as more or less sufficient to get your skills ready.

It's the same as for shoulder dystocia and we know that training models work very well for other obstetric situations like the shoulder dystocia. Which, of course, is an obstetric emergency and breech vaginal birth, it's a completely normal delivery. It is different but still you can train with these models and in courses very well.

A course for midwife addressing the same issues for supporting breech vaginal birth is something I really do support. And I do support courses combined obstetrician and midwives, because a labour ward on day-to-day work, midwives and obstetricians work together. So it is for me, absolutely mandatory to have training courses of both of the professionals combined together. And breech is a normal delivery, but it is something where we need to pay attention to several things. And I think the role of the midwife is to be there and to support normalcy.

Obstetricians tend to look at the things which are not going in the right direction and I think therefore it is very important that obstetrician and midwives look after women with the vaginal breech birth together. And the role of the midwife is to ensure normalcy. And that is important.

Vaginal breech birth—the ideal woman?

The question I believe, is there an ideal candidate for a breech vaginal delivery? And I can say, definitely, yes. Of course the woman who had previously uncomplicated vaginal birth is an ideal candidate for two reasons. First of all, we know when the previous delivery was for a term baby, which was normally grown, that her pelvis and her body is able to birth a baby. And that is very reassuring. And the second thing is that labour has already happened once and we know that in the second pregnancy and third pregnancies the delivery usually gets easier. So in a multiple breech vaginal delivery is something I always would support.

Of course you need to exclude obstetric reason for not having a vaginal birth. These are placenta praevia or fetal anomalies which are not able to be delivered vaginally. In general speaking, these things are all ruled out by the antenatal care and if the woman is healthy then I can't see any reason why not offering a woman who is in her first pregnancy a vaginal breech delivery. So even for primies it is a very important thing to offer the option of a vaginal breech delivery. While that, I do feel that a caesarean section for a breech baby is something we need to really be sure about. Because for her future life, if she's planning further pregnancies, that makes an impact. A caesarean section will lead to increased risk in all her future pregnancies. And therefore, I personally feel, women who are expecting their first babies should have the option to have a vaginal breech birth.

In many international guidelines, primies are always, like, looked at differently because as I said, women who had a previous vaginal birth, we know already that the woman is able to birth the baby. In a primi we don't know that and that's why people feel more uncomfortable. But I think because there are so important issues for the future life, it is important to concentrate on primies. In fact, in the unit where I used to work, 70% of all women were primies.

External cephalic version (ECV)

My views on external cephalic version is that it should be offered to all women. It is a safe procedure and it is successful in about 50% of all cases. The risks are minimal when you consider certain safeguards. Safeguards are that the woman is usually in the hospital and the baby will be monitored before, during and after the ECV: the external cephalic version. So it's a very safe procedure.

My personal view is that you should never try too hard. And because I'm an obstetrician having a lot of experience with vaginal breech births, I feel sometimes the baby has a reason. And then I offer it and if it doesn't work, I just encourage the woman to consider a vaginal breech delivery.

It is very important if you offer an external cephalic version that you don't talk about a failed external cephalic version, because the woman after that might feel, I have done something wrong or she might just blame herself.

So we should think about what words we use when we talk about breech babies. I usually don't say that the baby's in the wrong position, I say it's in a different position. And with the external cephalic version I think it is important if it's not successful then we should think about what do we offer the woman. And I think the next step then should be straight away to talk about vaginal breech delivery.

Advice for a woman with a breech presentation at 36 weeks' gestation?

My advice for a woman at 36 weeks of gestation coming with a breech presentation would be to really go to a clinic where there are experts in breech births. And that is usually a breech clinic. I would refer her to this clinic at 36 weeks because we need some time to talk about all the options to make a birth plan for the woman.

Now at 37 weeks, we usually consider external cephalic version as the first option which we offer to all women. If the external cephalic version is something the woman is not considering, then we talk about the option of a vaginal breech delivery. And there is, as well, the option of a planned caesarean section and I would usually recommend that for being able to make an informed choice, to really provide for all the options, enough information and even to give some written information and to make a second or even a third appointment to talk about the options and any questions.

So a breech clinic should address all these points and the appointments should be … there should be no time pressure, to talk to the woman and to the couple. Because it is very important that all the information is delivered and that the woman can really come to her own decision.

Alternative therapies

If a woman presents with a breech presentation and asked me about alternative methods, I usually encourage her to think about it. I think they are not harmful. And if the woman wants to try moxibustion or acupuncture, I think these are good options and I think they should be offered.

I personally think that because of all the issues which are coming up at some stage, like offering an external cephalic version, making a birth plan, vaginal breech delivery, caesarean section, we usually offer alternative methods prior to 36/37 weeks.

And up to then, the baby is still in breech position, I think it is important to prepare the woman. This baby is in a breech position and we need to think about what are the next steps. And I think that's important to allow her to go the way right from alternative methods and then thinking about the next steps if not successful.

Complications

Complications usually arise when people are nervous and have hands-on approach too quickly. And that leads to the problem that the baby, for example, there is a reflex, Moro reflex, that the baby for example gets the arms up and that can lead to extended arms and that can lead of course to a stuck baby.

So the training for obstetricians and midwives is always to be patient. Breech vaginal deliveries should be observed, rather than actively managed.

One of the things which I have studied over the last years is that the woman, when she is in upright position, that gravity helps to have a spontaneous vaginal breech birth, where you don't even need to have any kind of manoeuvres, no assistance, the baby delivers itself. So that is a really good thing because when you don't touch the baby, you don't risk any complications.

And one of the major safeguards is really to monitor the baby during the delivery and to be ready if there are any delays. And if there are any delays, you can help the baby to be delivered safely. And some of the skills which you need can be very well trained in courses. And that is something what I would usually support very much that people go to training courses for breech delivery.

Advice for midwives and midwifery students

Women who come for their 6-week postnatal appointment after a vaginal breech delivery are usually very happy and they are usually coming to say thank you. They feel that it was the right decision and they always like to come back personally to really give us their feedback, because obviously very often they are left alone with the decision of having a vaginal breech birth, by the friends and family. So usually what they find in the hospital or in the breech clinic, people supporting them to make an informed choice to come to the decision of having a vaginal breech birth. And usually we might be the first ones who support their wish and that's what they really appreciate.

If there is any advice I have for the students who look after women with a breech vaginal delivery, I would always like to point out that it is really important to support the woman in her choice, having a vaginal breech birth. Because very often they are left alone, and the family and friends, they usually don't understand why they have a vaginal breech delivery. So they feel very lonely and they sometimes feel even that they make a decision against the society. So I think as a midwife, as health professionals, we should really support the woman in her decision.

And that is something for a midwife, something what she can do all the time when she is with a woman during labour, giving her this support. And actually for me, it is really important as well that a breech delivery is a normal delivery. So I think it is important to make things normal and it is normal. And that is the support we should give these couples. And that they trust in their own ability to birth the baby out of this breech position.

And I think one of the major problems for the women is usually that they are left alone. Because everyone tells them, 'Why are you not having a caesarean?' And relatives, friends are putting a lot of pressure on these couples about, 'Why do you choose to have a vaginal breech delivery?' Because there is a lot of information out there which is actually not giving the true picture about vaginal breech delivery.

And we can prevent couples from taking this information on board of friends, relatives. So everyone looks on the internet and if you look up breech delivery, it's not helping. And therefore I think it's a very difficult decision and ours as professional health workers, we need to make sure that women feel supported.

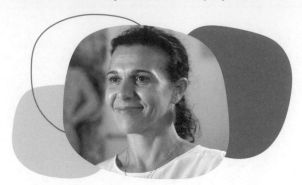

CHAPTER 3

Karolina

My name is Karol Petrovska, and I had a vaginal breech birth in March 2012. And I had a baby girl and it was a very straightforward birth, but the lead-up to it was fraught with anxiety and stress. And I look back now and it didn't have to be that way. So I'm happy to share my story so other women might, hopefully, and midwives and midwifery students, might learn from my experience.

Experience of being told your baby is in the breech position

I found out that Eden was in the breech position at 36 plus 5. And it was meant to be a routine antenatal appointment and my gorgeous midwife, who I'd known from booking in at 14 weeks, who I grew very, very fond of, was palpating my abdomen. And she said, 'I think this baby's still breech'.

And I remember a flurry of activity as she went out, got another midwife, got her to come back in, and she was palpating my abdomen. And my midwife was calling the obstetrician to try and book in an ECV. And I just remember feeling this rising heat and this anxiety just, it was a difficult, difficult appointment, was really stressful.

And they called in a registrar and we had to wait for him to become available. And he did an ultrasound and he confirmed it. He was really matter-of-fact about it which, when I look back now, it would have been nice for him to understand the weight of what he was telling me. And I don't think that he understood just how devastating it was for me to be there and to be hearing this.

I got a phone call from one of the midwives that I know very well. And she said, 'I've just spoken to an obstetrician at the Royal. He's waiting for your call. He's an expert in vaginal breech and he's waiting to hear from you'. I knew this obstetrician through work, so he knew who I was. And my response was, 'You have got to be kidding me'. That is for crazy hippies that have an issue with all birth intervention and I'm not going to risk my baby, blah, blah, blah. And I just thought she was crazy.

Accessing quality information on vaginal breech birth

In those few days between the diagnosis of the baby being breech and having an ECV, we went through a bit of a roller coaster ride and we spoke to a few people. But what was really helpful was watching some videos. We Googled some vaginal breech births and we tried to be judicious about which ones we chose.

And I remember turning to my husband and saying, 'What's the big deal? This is just a woman birthing a baby'. I mean I know it's bottom first, but she just pushed it out and her body did all the work. Like you do when it's a cephalic presenting baby.

And so that was really powerful. The video was really powerful because it normalised it. And I had initially thought, oh my goodness, they're going to have their legs up on the table and they're going to be pulling this baby out. And it was completely wrong and completely off. I don't know where I got that idea from. It's, you know, it's the hysteria that surrounds vaginal breech birth, I think. And I'm not a maternity clinician. I haven't witnessed any, you know, vaginal breech births, so the video was powerful.

And speaking with clinicians that are about the age of 40 or 45, that were practising before the vaginal breech, the Term Breech Trial, was released in 2000. And speaking with them, they would say to me before the Term Breech Trial, it was just another way a baby came out and it's actually quite straightforward. But if the baby needs some help getting out, there are things that you can do. But it's not that different to the manoeuvres that you might do for shoulder dystocia. It's the same kind of thing.

The next thing that I did was look at the Term Breech Trial and the analyses, the subsequent analyses of the Term Breech Trial. And I realised when you really pick it apart, it's just a really bad study that … where the conclusions aren't justified.

Because I had an option and because I had clinicians that would support me in that option, I still remained in the centre of this pregnancy and this process of having this baby. And when the doors closed, and you just don't have any options, you're on the outside and the system's putting itself in the centre saying, 'This is how we manage you'.

The ECV didn't turn the baby because the baby didn't want to be turned. And she was firmly wedged in a frank breech position. She'd been there since, I don't know, she must have liked the position for some reason.

So I rang the obstetrician at the Royal Hospital for Women and I said, 'When can we come and see you?' He made himself available and he presented the facts. And what sealed the deal was he said, 'With a skilled clinician, the risks', which he did talk about, 'the risks are about the same as a caesarean section. Not exactly, but it's pretty close'. And given that I had a 5-hour first labour and birth, he said, 'I don't want to minimise labour and birth, but you'll probably cough this baby out'.

And that was really powerful, why wouldn't you give it a go? They are very clear in saying the first sign of any distress and it's an emergency caesar, no mucking around, we're not going to … and that was really powerful too. They weren't these cowboys that were just trying to, you know, do some underground thing. This was an evidence-based approach and the risks were clearly laid out. And he gave me about an 80% success rate. It was a guesstimate, but I asked him, can you give me a guesstimate? It's pretty good odds, so that's what sealed the deal. That's what really … we walked out of there saying, yeah, let's give it a go.

So when we left the hospital, we didn't really think about the influences that might make us doubt our decision.

Social discourse on vaginal breech birth

There were still 3 weeks to go and a lot of damage was done by other people in that 3 weeks. And what it made me realise was that other people feel very strongly about what women should do with their bodies when they're pregnant and having a baby. I kind of see the forces, the political forces, the views of society, as a real violation of women's human rights when they're pregnant. It's my body, this is my choice. I feel like I've made an informed choice.

But when I did share my thoughts about what our decision was with some friends, I got heavily judged for that. And anything that I would try and say, I would just look like I was one of those crazy, risk-takers. I think it's up to the system to understand and accommodate women instead of looking at them like they are baby killers, which I know happens.

So we decided to not tell anybody else, except for my mum. She was really happy that we had the option to try for a vaginal breech birth. And she knew that I knew people in the system and that I had made a sound decision.

So that familial interaction was really quite positive, but friends, not so positive. And so we decided not to tell my husband's family, and kind of cocoon ourselves. And I think that's really sad. I think that's a missed opportunity to raise the profile of vaginal breech. I think that is a missed opportunity to get excited about the impending arrival of a baby.

I found keeping quiet, really sad. That was the way we managed it though and that was the best decision that we could make at the time, I think, based on the circumstances and our experiences.

I had to ban myself from the internet because there are no, very few, good news stories about vaginal breech. There are distorted stories, there are people judging, there are really negative experiences to be had on the internet about vaginal breech birth.

So I sort of developed a real passion for how social discourse impacts on women's decision making for vaginal breech birth. Because there's not enough good evidence-based information out there; I mean it doesn't always work out, but this is about keeping your options open and staying at the centre of the process.

Experience of having a vaginal breech birth

I got to 40 plus 1 and the contractions were about 3 minutes apart, and we called the hospital—that was about 5 pm. And we went in there and they did a vaginal examination and I was 7 cm. And I laboured for a couple of hours. And it was just normal labour, it was pretty straightforward.

I remember one thing that made me feel really good was even though it was the birthing suite, it was a clinical environment, there was a lamp there, that was this really homey kind of second-hand looking lamp that I think they try to bring in to try and mimic a birth centre. And all the lights went off and they just put this lamp on. It was really soft light and it was lovely. It didn't have this glaring, kind of artificial thing, you know, going on. And I just remember thinking that's so nice. It's such a small thing but it was really nice.

And about 2 hours after we got in there, I felt like I had to push, I really felt the need to push. So they got me on the bed and did another vaginal examination and stretched me; I was fully dilated. And they led me to the birthing stool, which I had been told that that's what I had to sit on. That's how they do vaginal breech births at this hospital. I know a lot of women like the stool because they're upright. But it wasn't the stool that I didn't like, it was being told that that was my only option.

And the obstetrician, though, he was really good. He kept calling it. He kept saying, 'Okay, I felt the bottom when it came down; it's just gone back up again. It'll probably stay down the next time'.

There are people in the room that wanted to see it. So there was a bit of a cast of thousands there, which I was fine about; they'd asked me and I was fine. I knew the importance of clinicians needing to see it. But they were cheering and it was so nice. It was so, so nice, it was so … it worked. It really worked, it really sort of spurred me on.

And the other thing was one of the midwives said, 'How about I hold up a mirror so you can see what you're doing?' And that was really powerful. And I know that's normal and I know that happens all the time, mirrors come out all the time. But, wow, I saw this bum appear and I didn't see that the first time with my daughter. I was in the bath tub, I was lying down. It was a great water birth but I couldn't see what was going on. So to see yourself pushing this bottom out was so powerful. So the mirror was very, very, very helpful. So I would encourage that mirror to come out where you can, for all the student midwives watching this video.

And then at each push, the obstetrician would call what was happening and that was so helpful. 'Legs are out. Another push, right shoulder's out, another push.'

I had to get that head out, I really knew I had to get that head out. And it came out in a couple of pushes. He didn't need to help her come out, she kind of did just slide out and it was very straightforward and pretty amazing. And she was fine.

She went pink and she started crying and everyone was cheering. And it was a great, great birth; it was a very positive experience.

Reflections following a vaginal breech birth

I didn't really get a chance to debrief about my birth experience to the extent that I wanted to. And I don't know that many women do in clinical settings, because everybody's so busy.

And I think the way that I've chosen to process the anxiety and the stress leading up to it is to go back and study. And it is to speak at conferences to clinicians and to women. That is my way of unpacking a lot of stress and anxiety in those 3 weeks leading up to it.

I think the way that I've debriefed about it is to continue to talk about it in some of these circumstances and to study the effects that the negativity and the anxiety that other people put on women in this position. I think that we need to shine a light on that. It doesn't have to be that way.

This was essentially a very normal birth. We're put in this really difficult position and we have to navigate this at this really vulnerable time in our lives. And it shouldn't be that way; it's just another way for a baby to come out.

Advice for midwives caring for women with a breech presentation

My advice would be to try and keep the woman at the centre of this experience. The system will try and push her out to the edge and put itself in the centre. If you can, if you know how your maternity networks work, if you don't offer vaginal breech birth at the hospital that you're working at as a midwife when you graduate, get to know where she can go. She shouldn't be the one navigating the system. You need to be able to be ready to provide that information for her.

If she wants a caesarean after she's had all the information and all the evidence then keep her at the centre and support her. If she wants to have a vaginal breech birth or try, help her get to where she needs to go. It may be that she lives in a rural area and she needs to go to a metropolitan hospital. Is there any way that you can facilitate that? Are there people that you know through your networks that you can contact to facilitate that transfer?

I think it's really easy to forget about postnatal care because it's a vaginal breech birth. But it's so important. Please not just concentrate on the fact that she's having a vaginal breech birth. But the woman needs to have the opportunity to talk about management of the third stage.

CHAPTER 4

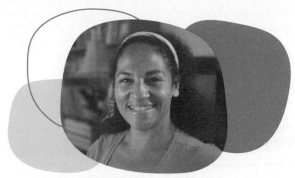

Malika's story

My name's Malika and I have three children. I had my first child when I was 28 and I had my third child when I was 41.

Having a baby over 40 years of age

I would have much preferred to have had my own midwife. I know some women go into the midwife scheme and get to have one midwife or two that look after them. And I would have loved that, especially after 40, especially with having had such great births the first two times. I thought I would have been a good candidate for being at home or having a homebirth but there was a little bit of pressure, being over 40, to go to the hospital.

My partner pushed for more tests because of my age and I felt a strong push from the ultrasound clinic and the obstetrician, is that right, who was on to have all these tests done because of my age. But I trusted my gut feeling that I was fine and that with the blood test results were so positive that I wouldn't get them done. I didn't want to have the extra testing. So I stood my ground; it's my body and I said no. And everything was fine.

I was positive for strep, so they weren't happy about that because of my age, I guess. And because of the strep they didn't want me, I wasn't eligible to have a homebirth. And then when the baby was born they felt that they needed to do tests on him because of the strep, straight away. They didn't know; it's interesting because with the first two births I was never tested for that, so it wasn't an issue.

How did my body get back together after having a baby over 40? It was fine actually. I think I learnt a lot after the first one where I ate far too many cinnamon rolls after I gave birth and didn't exercise a lot. And it took a long time to get back to being healthy. I was in my 20s. So I'd learnt by the 40s to just eat moderately, don't eat for two when you're pregnant, just eat for one and keep exercising. And after the baby was born, yeah, just gentle exercises, moving around, getting out of the house and just, it's hard to remember. It is a bit of a blur when you give birth, but I don't think that it was any harder to get back to my body shape after 40.

Continuity of care

I actually found the communication not that great because you're always seeing a different person and they're so busy. The hospital antenatal clinic was so busy, always running late, and I think they were just in-out-in-out. They just sort of did the basic tests and the basic checks and go.

Ideally, I would have had a consistency of care with one or several midwives who knew my history and who knew me and who knew what my wishes were. And I think if that had happened with each birth, would have been smoother and easier and could have been even more positive experiences. Certainly with the last birth, it would have been a more positive experience.

Having a baby taken to the special care nursery

So when Jesse was born, it was all quite a shock to my system literally. He was kind of whisked away by the midwife and she felt concerned that he was pale from the waist down and didn't know why. And I felt like that was all such a blur and it all happened so fast. I didn't get a chance to hold Jesse, I didn't get a chance to look at him, or look in his eyes. And he was whisked away before I could even say, 'I don't want him to have antibiotics. Can we just wait for an hour or two? And just see if his colour comes good?'

So I felt like it was really taken out of my hands. And once he was into the system and they said, 'Right, he's on antibiotics. He has to be on antibiotics for 48 hours while we do tests and before we can let him go'. And so within that hour after his birth, he was in the system of the 'better safe than sorry'. And I do have a friend who's a doctor who said, 'Well, you want to be better safe than sorry. If something went wrong, you'd be angry and saying "Why didn't you do something?"'

In this case, there was nothing wrong with him, but it took over an hour for me to hold my baby and to look at him and to breastfeed him. And they wanted to keep him in the neonatal ward overnight and I had to kind of demand, very firmly, that 'No, he seems fine in all respects. I want him to be with me on the ward'. And so when they called around and went, 'Okay, he can be with you, but you have to bring him back every couple of hours to be given more antibiotics'. So all through the night I had to wake him up and take him down to the neonatal ward to be given more drugs. And then after 48 hours was told there was nothing wrong, he was fine, he could go home.

The first time I saw my baby he was strapped up with a cannula, 'Welcome to the world; here, have a couple of needles'. He had his harness, baby harness, monitor on, heart monitor on him. And he was in a humidicrib and he just looked so little and it was … it was my baby. Whereas I know from the other two births, where I was able to just hold them straight away.

I loved holding my babies. So I missed that. I missed having that skin-to-skin contact and that, being able to hold him straight away. But I understand that if they have to go to the neonatal ward, then they have to go. And you do anything to have your baby be happy and well.

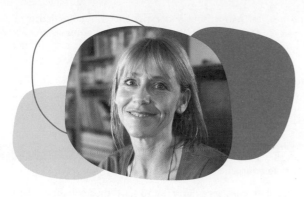

CHAPTER 5

Emma's story

I'm Emma, I'm 44 years old. I have seven children. I have five girls and two boys. My eldest daughter is 16½ and my youngest is 9 months.

Having seven children

I like the idea of the continued midwife where you have the same midwife from the start of your pregnancy through to labour. But I know there's only limited spots on that program and so I felt that it's probably better for women who are on their first child or who need it more than me, who haven't had an easy time of labour and pregnancy, to use one of those spaces.

So I've just gone with the shared care program; seems to be the easiest. I can go and see my GP or go and see the midwives at the midwife clinic, and have a few appointments in the hospital where you always have to wait such a long time. So try and keep those appointments to the minimum.

I was told that I could haemorrhage so they had to put a cannula in my hand, which wasn't very pleasant, in case they needed to treat me quickly if I haemorrhaged after giving birth. I was also told that sometimes the contractions aren't as effective because I've stretched so many times. That my body might find it hard to have effective contractions that will actually push a baby out.

I think that I was also told about the risks because of my age, but once you've jumped through those hurdles and had the tests along the way, that felt okay. I didn't particularly feel concerned, I just felt that things were going to be okay. I don't remember feeling worried that I might haemorrhage. I felt well, I felt healthy, I always felt the babies move. And I've always had my babies in hospital, and so I haven't been concerned that I wouldn't be able to get hospital treatment quickly if needs be.

I know a few other people who've had lots of babies and haven't necessarily had problems.

I think I just felt … my body knew what to do and they'd all been fine up until now. Healthy babies, spring back into shape easily, quickly. My body seemed to know what it was meant to be doing and has always done what it's meant to do reasonably well.

In terms of body shape, I kind of spring back fairly quickly. But I've got veins on my legs from, I think number four onwards, which get a little bit worse with each child. Nothing that an injection can't sort out when I've stopped breast-feeding. And, don't have stretch marks but have some sort of looser skin on my tummy. But, really it's the story of my life so that's kind of the way it's going to be.

Labour progression in a grand multipara

In some of the later babies, the contractions started and then seemed to stop, which might have been related to me having more babies. But the contractions … actually, the final contractions didn't seem like they were as bad as they were in earlier pregnancies. I actually got to 10 cm and remember being quite surprised that the pain hadn't been as bad as I thought it was going to be, to get to 10 cm.

I think one of the good things is when you're ready, when you're ready for the baby, when everything is sorted at home, then you'll be ready to have the baby.

I remember I had my daughter's birthday, got that out of the way, then she had a sleepover, we had a party. The next day I went into labour. So I think me being ready in my head and everything being right at home, that has been one of the things that the midwives have said. I think there's a lot of psychological stuff with having a baby that you don't necessarily realise.

Reflections about midwifery care from a grand multipara

One of the things I find with midwives is that they need to listen to you and some of them listen more than others.

There's a few qualities that I found that I like in some of the midwives and I've had some really lovely, wonderful midwives. And the ones that have been particularly good for me are the ones that listen and act accordingly, rather than just appearing to listen but not really. The ones that are kind but not patronising and experienced but not jaded or cynical or domineering, because they think they know. Calm, so even if things don't go to plan or aren't going as quickly as anticipated, they stay calm and that helps you feel calm and makes you feel that you don't need to worry, everything's in control.

It's nice when midwives guide you and maybe make suggestions but not in a bossy way. Sometimes midwives do need to tell you exactly what needs to be done. They need to … with one of my children, I had to lie on my side because the head was positioned in a way that he wasn't going to come out very easily. So she needed to get him to rotate so that she could help him come out. She just needed to tell me what to do, which she did very nicely, very kindly, and it worked. And he came out very easily after that.

Midwives are an advocate for mums and babies, and sometimes they need to talk to the doctors and will … sometimes they need to talk to the husbands. But you need to know they're on your side and they want the best for you and baby.

It's about having the balance. I think for some midwives, it probably comes very naturally to have those qualities. And for some midwives, it's some skills they need to learn, about respecting the mum and staying calm, being experienced, being kind.

The social side of having lots of children

One of the things that's made it hard having a large family is that we have no family support in Australia. We're both, my husband and I are from the UK, and all our family are still in the UK. Of course, we have a large circle of friends and they help and they are kind of like family to us now. But our children hopefully won't have that lack of family. Hopefully there's a lot of them; they'll have their nieces, nephews, cousins, grandparents. We'll be around, so they will enjoy that large family, even as they get older.

One of the other difficult things is that my career really has had to be put on hold since I had my first. I went back very briefly before I had my third and that was quite a juggle. And since then I haven't gone back to work and I did have quite a nice career before I had children, which I hope one day I will get back to.

On the plus side and what's made it easy to have a large family, I think is, we have … since my husband started working locally—he runs his own business—so he's much more flexible than he used to be when he was working in Sydney. He can … like he's looking after my little boy at the moment, he's taken him to playgroup. He can come along to the school events and if for any reason I can't, he'll be there at assembly, watching the assembly item or watching an award being given out.

And friends, of course, they help out. They bring us meals when we've had a baby and things like that. So a very supportive community we have here. And financial stability really, that helps. We own our own home. I think having seven children costs a lot of money and so finances are tighter than they would be if we just had two. But thankfully, we're okay.

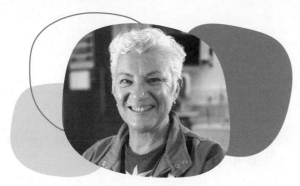

CHAPTER 6

Jane's story

Hi, I'm Jane. I'm a midwife who has worked in a rural, remote area for the last 2 years. Our local hospital was a non-birthing unit and the women had to travel at least 400 km to have their baby, but we provided antenatal and postnatal care there.

Birth in a rural setting

The main difference between birthing in a rural, remote area and the urban area is the fact that the women have to leave their homes up to a month before the birth. And this incorporates so many problems for them. Where do they go? Which hospital do they choose to have their baby? How do they get there? Where do they stay when they get there? And there's that pressure once they get there, that it's costing them to stay there.

So, then they have to think about when am I going to have this baby? And so if they are offered an induction or they request an induction or caesarean, for them, that's a good option. Because they know when they're going to have their baby. Then their partner can come and join them because usually they have to stay wherever they live and work until the baby comes.

And for the women where I was, it was a 4-hour drive to the nearest place to have a baby. And so if they just went into labour normally, then they'd have to call their partner and say, 'Quick, get here now'. And so I think there's a lot of pressure to get on and have the baby. Whereas in the city, I think women when they're worried about getting to the hospital in time, it was half an hour at the most that they'd be travelling.

And so that was the main issue that I found with the women out there, is the distance. It's just … it puts so much pressure on them. And I know, you're less likely to go into labour naturally if you're worrying about when you're going to go into labour, and whether your partner's going to get there and what's happening to your other children. And those sorts of things are much more important to those women.

They weren't worried about what sort of a birth it was going to be. They weren't focused on the experience like urban women, much more focused on a feel-good experience, if you can say that about birth. In the country it's much more practical: How am I going to get there? How long's it gonna take? When will I get home? How much is it gonna cost me?

Leaving town to give birth

I guess one of the big issues, particularly for the Indigenous women where I was, is the fact that they often have quite a few other children. Or they're quite young and so they need, or they feel they need, more support from their mother or their sisters. And so what it does, is it breaks up families around a time when your family should be around you. And so they're having to leave partners and other children behind. Who's going to look after those children? What's the partner going to get up to? Is he going to actually come for the birth or not?

And for the Indigenous women, they just don't have any money. Often, 'Oh, I can't go down this week because I don't get paid until Monday, so I can't go down before Monday'. And then the bus doesn't go on Tuesday. It only goes Monday, Wednesday, Friday. So there's a lot of issues around transport as well as accommodation. And just separating families.

The Aboriginal women don't birth in the bush. And they were very urban where I was, but many of them would just stay home. You would see them at an antenatal appointment and I would say, 'You really need to be getting yourself out of town for this birth'. And, 'Oh yes, yes, yes, I'll go, I'll go. My sister will take me tomorrow'. And then you would see her 3 days later still in town.

So often the births that we did have there were women in labour, rocking up, well established, and we'd be on the phone getting the air ambulance to take them out of town. And more often than not, they would end up having their baby before the plane got there. And yes, so that was their way of not going away. You'd just ignore it. They knew the babies would come. They knew, particularly with the two midwives in town, that there were people, and there were two doctors while I was there, with obstetrics. So they were fairly confident that they would have experienced staff looking after them.

The problem was that we, the midwives in particular, were only working Monday to Friday 9 to 5 and so we weren't on call for births. And we got a lot of pressure not to encourage women to stay in town. If they turned up in labour it was our fault because we hadn't made them leave town. I don't know how you make people leave town if they don't want to, but.

Inductions, caesareans, are seen as a good thing because it gives them a date and a time when that baby's gonna come. And so they can organise their lives, the rest of their lives around that. The accommodation is limited. I mean it's hard even if they can get to stay with family, it's hard staying with people for an extended period of time. Even if you love them dearly, you're not in your own space. You don't have your things around you, you feel awkward and not knowing how long that's gonna be.

Working in a rural community town as a midwife

It was a small country town, 3000 people. And there was a multipurpose health service there. So it was like a little country hospital. And it had a birthing room and it was well stocked. One of the reasons I went there was that I thought that we were going to be … going to do birthing. And when I looked at the room I thought, I can work here. We had a beautiful triangular bath in the corner just like the birth centre in the city. I thought, 'yeah, we can have babies here'. Unfortunately, it didn't ever get started. So they would come in, we would look after them. We even had a CTG if we needed that. We had all the resus equipment, we had everything you could need.

So we would just go about looking after them until the air ambulance got there. And then we would hand over. They'd be flown out. Usually, there was this unwritten rule that if they were 5 cm or less, they would be flown out. If they were beyond that, then they'd stay and have the baby and then they would be flown out.

The good things about working in that area was that it was a small community. And so I would often see the women when I was in the local supermarket or in the post office. I would see them after they'd had their babies and see the babies growing up. That was lovely. We had quite a bit of continuity. The women would, once they got to know that there were midwives that they could see, they would come and see us regularly. So I got some continuity.

The bad part about that was that they would leave town at least 2 or 3 weeks before the baby was due, and they would probably stay away for a week or two afterwards. So there was this huge gap between, say, 36 weeks and 2 weeks postnatal where I wouldn't see them or know what had happened, sometimes. 'Cause some of them would go quite a long way away out of our area health service so I had no contact. And then they would come back. There would sometimes be breastfeeding issues that I felt if I had been there at the birth and been able to follow them through afterwards, may not have developed.

And sometimes they wouldn't even make contact afterwards, so I'd lose that. When I was working in the city and I was working caseload, I had that beautiful continuity right through from beginning to 2 or 3 weeks postnatal.

For the women, I think, it was really hard. They'd build up this relationship with us during their pregnancy. Then they'd have to go somewhere else to have their baby and give birth with strangers. And for me, as a midwife, a lot of what I do in an antenatal visit is education. But I found it really hard because I didn't know where she was going to have her baby or how they would treat her there, what their policies were generally.

I noticed the nearest hospital, the number of women that had pethidine when they were somewhere between 5 and 10 cm, often 7 cm; a multi having pethidine at that point, to me, it's just pointless. All you're going to do is knock your baby out and not give the woman good pain relief.

So trying to work around that and give her some skills to achieve what she wanted in her birth. But as I said earlier, the women often weren't so focused on their birth experience, it was just, 'When am I going to have my baby?' That was more important than how it was going to be born and what they were going to do in labour.

And the things that I felt would help them in labour, often the midwives looking after them weren't of the same mindset. And so they would be encouraging them to have pain relief, epidurals, narcotics, rather than getting in the shower or the bath, which is what I would have suggested.

They were often kept on the bed and monitored; what was, in my opinion, unnecessary monitoring. All seemed to have an admission CTG, whether there were indications for that or not, and we all know that's really one of the first interventions. They'll find something wrong and keep that monitor on, keep the woman on the bed. So, yeah, the cascade would happen. But the women didn't seem to be too upset about that. Because they didn't know that it could be different, I guess.

High-risk women

High-risk women were a huge issue for us, particularly the Indigenous women because, I mean they have lots of problems. Diabetes is rife. They would often have small babies; there's a lot of smoking, there's quite a bit of drugs and alcohol issues in that area. To get them seen by even a registrar was quite difficult.

In theory we had a registrar come out once a month, but particularly over the Christmas break, last November he came out and he didn't come again until March, end of March. So it's a huge gap. And in that time, I can remember many times trying to get women seen in the nearest large centre was quite difficult. Mainly transport, getting them there. We'd often make appointments, try and organise some transport.

There was one woman I remember in particular. We organised transport, they turned up and they had to get there at 6 o'clock in the morning to pick her up. They get there, they went to the wrong house. They didn't ever find her. So we arranged for the next day and then she wasn't available. And it just went on and on, trying to get her seen was almost impossible.

They really need to have an outreach service. But it's not a regular thing. I mean, it's quite expensive for the health service to provide that. And I think, often it's seen as, we'll get the women to come to us and that gets rid of this huge cost to our health service. But, yes, to get them seen was a huge problem and often they would end up not being seen until very late in the pregnancy.

When they have diabetes, you can't just send them off to see the dietitian or the endocrinologist. We didn't have those people in town, so then they had to go at least 400 km to access those services. And even when they did, then they would come back and their diet wasn't great. I don't know how well they actually controlled their diabetes. Yeah, there were quite a lot of issues around high-risk pregnancies. And I don't know whether some of them actually understood what our concerns were. That and how it would affect their babies.

We did see a lot of growth restriction, or should I say growth-restricted babies, for various reasons. And even with those women, things like getting an ultrasound could be an issue. We had two ultrasonographers in town, but just recently, both of them were out of town. And trying to get the ultrasound done before the women actually got to the main centre was sometimes impossible.

So it felt like we were chasing our tails a lot of the time, trying to get services that we take for granted in the city. Even blood tests sometimes would take much longer because they'd have to be sent out of town to be done. They could do the basic stuff but a lot of the other things would have to be sent away.

Yes, there were a number of women that I cared for at some stage during their pregnancy who did not access any real antenatal care. Most of them would have an early ultrasound or an ultrasound at 20 weeks. They thought that 20-week ultrasound was when you found out what sex your baby was. So sometimes we would have a clear idea of when that baby was due, but often we didn't.

And we would often have women who would just turn up in labour, having not seen anybody throughout their pregnancy. And that was really hard, very hard to know even where to start and what you needed to do for that woman.

Fortunately, we didn't have too many bad outcomes, but it was very difficult to care for women who didn't have antenatal care. I mean, you don't know whether they have diabetes or whether this baby is growth restricted or whether there are any other issues. And so you're not sure what's going to happen when she does give birth.

The importance of the community around birth

I guess, as a midwife, I really see birth as a social event, not necessarily a medical event. There are, of course, some women who develop complications and they need to be transferred out. But to me, it seems wrong that you can't have your family around you when you have your baby, that the local town don't find out until a week later that you've had your baby. They don't get to see your baby when it's newborn. And people want to do that.

We had a young woman who had a 26-weeker and we had to wait. She actually gave birth in the hospital, and we were waiting on NETS for three hours. In that time, I think nearly every young, Indigenous woman in town came in and saw that baby. And it was just beautiful to watch the social interaction around the birth of this baby and the support the young mother got. And then she had to leave and it was months before she came back to town. A lot of people, even her own mother was trying to find a way to get to Sydney to be with her. Huge issues around that sort of thing. And I think that's one of the saddest things about it, is that it breaks up families, rather than bringing them together. Which, in the city, that's how it seems, that all these families come together when a baby is born. Whereas up there, it tears them apart.

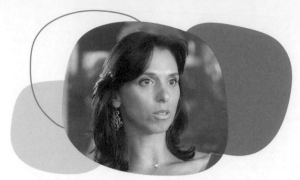

CHAPTER 7

Melanie's story

My name is Melanie. I am 6 months pregnant with number two. My son, Jake, was born 2 years ago exactly, and I'll be telling you my story about that.

Deciding to have an elective caesarean

So I have to start the story by saying that having Jake was quite a journey. He was difficult to come by. We had him through IVF and that really influenced my decision as to how to have him. We did a little bit of reading, a bit of research and spoke to professionals on the whole, rather than friends, because we quickly realised that there's a bit of a stigma out there about birth; caesarean, natural, whatever it may be.

And through my reading and my research, I found that, it's probably … it looked like it was a safer option for the baby to have a caesarean delivery. I was very nervous about it. I can't say that it was an easy decision. I had worked with someone previously who had a caesarean delivery and had an epidural. And she actually became paralysed. Now, I don't know how connected the two were, what the issue was, but it stuck in my mind. And giving birth was a scary cloud that really hovered above the whole pregnancy.

And then we met our obstetrician. One of the reasons we chose him was because we knew that if we opted to have a caesarean, he would do it. He wouldn't talk us out of it. And that's exactly how it was.

I still wanted to talk it through. He didn't sway me either way. But he was quite clear with the benefits or the negatives and he just laid the cards on the table and said, 'This is how it is and feel free to do a bit more research. And we can talk about it at subsequent appointments'.

I have family members in the business and the doctor in the family had written a very in-depth article about what a caesarean actually entails. So I had a look at that, which was quite scary, I have to say. Because you think of having a baby as having a baby. You don't think of it as being a serious operation. And it is a serious operation and a lot can go wrong. So the article was eye-opening, to say the least. He was very clear about what can happen, to do with the pain or the recovery. But that was a good starting point because it was very clear.

I spent some time talking to women who'd had caesareans, not too many. Because once I make my mind about something, I kind of go ahead and just relax into it and just let it happen. So the experiences that I heard were all very positive and I also decided to meet with the anaesthetist that we had booked in for the caesarean. So we met with him probably 2 months before we had Jake. And he talked me through it. He very quickly realised how nervous I was.

Giving birth to Jake

The day before the caesarean, we met with the anaesthetist. He booked us in and he gave us the little pads which were the local anaesthetic that Neil was to put on my back, at 5 o'clock in the morning, 'cause we were having Jake at 8 or 8.30. I wasn't allowed to eat a lot of food after midnight. I did wake up at 5 and have a cup of tea and a piece of toast. And we stuck the anaesthetic onto my back.

So we drove into hospital. Neil had to go into the reception area. I was taken upstairs into my room and gowned up. And then the anaesthetist came to get me. And Neil met me in the room off the theatre. I was nervous. I was cold, I remember always being cold, I'm always cold in theatre.

And that's part of the nerves I guess, as well. I got some of the, I think they call it the 'Michael Jackson drug', that relaxed me a little bit. And it took effect quite quickly. I could feel that things were just … it just took the edge off for me. And to be honest, I can't imagine doing it without it; it just helped me.

And then the epidural was inserted. I remember hearing the little … there's like a little air break that you hear during the injection. But I couldn't feel a thing. I was quite surprised at how relaxed I was at that stage. And then I was in theatre.

The one thing that surprised me about the whole process, really, was the amount of people who were in the theatre. There was our obstetrician and our anaesthetist who I'd met before. Then there was an assisting obstetrician. And then there were, I think, three or four nurses or midwives milling around. And I didn't expect that. So, yeah, that was a surprise.

I didn't feel that my privacy was invaded. I felt safe. It didn't bother me, I knew that they were there for a reason. It's a hospital, everybody knows their role. I couldn't see a lot either because I had, the screen was up on my tummy. So I guess that also makes it a bit more of an intimate setting. And Neil was by my side and the anaesthetist was by my side, taking photos. And he liked to joke a bit, so that was a bit of a light relief. It just all happened so quickly, it was amazing.

The obstetrician just stated that he was cutting. And the next thing I knew is I heard Jake cry. And the next thing, he was on my ... oh, there was also a paediatrician in the room, so that was another professional. Yeah the next thing, Jake was on my chest and we did request to have skin-to-skin.

It was very important to us and we were aware that there were some doctors who didn't particularly like it, because the theatre is quite cool. So they tend to wrap the babies quite quickly. But we asked for that not to happen. So he was on me for quite a while, probably about half an hour or so, while I was being sewn up. And again, that felt like it just went so quickly, it was just amazing.

The next thing I knew, I was in the recovery room. Now Jake wasn't allowed to come into the recovery room with me because it is a general hospital. So he was with Neil. And I was actually really pleased that we got that opportunity, not to be separated, but more for Jake to spend that skin-on-skin time with Neil. And I think Neil really enjoyed it.

So then I was wheeled back into my room and saw Jake on Neil and it was just lovely. And the moment he came back onto my chest, it was just bliss. I'm going to cry.

Having the midwife there was priceless for that first half-hour or so. But just having someone who's done this before, with us, and obviously Jake wasn't having any milk yet, but just to get the whole ball rolling, get us settled, comfortable, know how to hold him properly, even though he wasn't such a little baby. It was great to have that third person in the room.

I think we were so excited that by 10 o'clock, I was back in the room. We'd had Jake at 8:30. I think it took us, maybe by lunchtime, we started making calls and letting people know. I was tired but it wasn't going to be overcome by having a sleep that kind of tired. It was more an emotional elation and a relief, an absolute relief that he was there.

Establishing breastfeeding

So I was alone in the room. Jake was taken to the nursery, which is just a godsend, I have to say. For the first two nights, he slept in the nursery. I remember the nurses coming to wake me to feed him in the middle of the night at some stage, I think it was early morning. He was crying so that pacified him quite quickly.

We were transferred to the hotel on day 3 and I remember that night, I was actually walking the room with Jake because he wouldn't settle. And I think that was probably a sign that there was a break between the colostrum and the milk coming in. And it was quite lovely because there were a few other couples who arrived that day. And you could hear from the far away rooms, babies crying in the middle of the night. So we were all in the same boat.

But he settled after a few hours and had a good sleep, and I had a good sleep, and then Neil arrived in the morning. And the breastfeeding kind of happened. We did build a relationship with the lactation consultant before we had Jake. I went to a talk by a lady and then decided that we probably should get her number and keep it going.

And she came to visit us in hospital, and then we made an appointment to see her while we were in the hotel. And that was very, very helpful. She just made sure that what I was doing was right and gave me a few tips. Nothing more than that. I think we were lucky that Jake was taking to the breast quite easily. It was comfortable to me, it was comfortable for him. Yeah, it all went quite smoothly.

What did happen to us is that we got home 6 days after the caesarean and the next day I was experiencing difficulties with the feeding. So we very quickly called her again and saw her. And she gave us a few tips and that was it and we were on the road to success.

I breastfed Jake for 5 months. I lost a lot of weight very quickly from the breastfeeding. I actually gained about 11 or 12 kg in my pregnancy, but lost about 15 or 16 kg once I had him. So it was quite drastic. My hair was falling out also, about month 4, I lost a lot of hair, and my family doctor suggested maybe weaning him. So by 6 months, he was only on the breast once a day. And I kept that going, early morning feed, I kept that going until he was 1, and then was quite happy to give that away.

I felt that the midwives were very supportive and they were all there for the same outcome. But sometimes it was too much and the advice that they were giving me was conflicting. And it was up to me to wade through the information and to make a decision as to what worked for me. Which wasn't easy in the first few days; hence, the lactation consultant was quite helpful. Once we got to the hotel, I felt that the midwives there were possibly more confident and more experienced, and maybe read me better. And also let me be, a little bit. And they had confidence in my confidence, if that's possible at such an early stage.

So I only saw the midwife at the hotel, maybe, twice a day; one of those was to get my injection. At the hospital, it was a different story. There was someone coming into the room quite often and checking on me and making sure that things were happening. But again, the information was conflicting at times.

Early parenting

The first 2 days I couldn't get out of bed; I was still attached to the epidural port. So it was quite cumbersome. On the third day I got out of bed to have my shower. It wasn't comfortable, but it wasn't horrific. I also didn't really suffer a gush of blood or any of that. So I think everything was happening mildly, not too terrible.

I do recall an incident where I felt uncomfortable. And it was on the third day, it was the morning of the third day. I had to get out of bed to have a shower. And that was quite daunting because it was the first time I was actually going to stand on my feet.

And a midwife, a young midwife, had come into the room. And she was sitting on the chair, helping me, instructing me what to do. And also warning me that having my first shower and there'll be blood and all the usual things. But I felt that I was being, maybe, talked at, rather than talked to, and explained and taught what to do. I was nervous about the process. Luckily it was all fine and straightforward, but I felt uneasy in the whole scene.

What helped me was probably more me than her. I needed to have a shower. I needed to put on some makeup. I needed to be me again. Neil wasn't in the room so it wasn't that I looked at him and sought some comfort in him. I just got on and did it. Admittedly, I think now, I look back at it and think, that's what a mother is, you just get on and do it.

It was probably the one point where I felt quite vulnerable in the whole experience. And I just got up and did it, but I didn't feel very supported.

I do remember sneezing or coughing and that was sore, but nothing out of the ordinary. I was comfortable getting in the car on day 3 to go to the hotel. I was comfortable, I was confident and I felt safe being in a room on my own. I wasn't scared. My wound was clean. What I did do is, my obstetrician recommended putting a pad above the wound, so that it would protect it from any pants I was wearing. So I was wearing actually a maternity pad under my underpants, just to have a barrier. Which was over and above the bandages that were on there.

Having a bath was fine. I didn't feel that I was being stopped from doing anything I needed to do. We went downstairs to the lobby to have a coffee. I walked around. We went into the nurses' room to give Jake his first bath and I was part of that. So my mobility came back very soon after; within 48 hours I was fine. Carrying Jake was comfortable, carrying him in the capsule was comfortable, sitting in a car. It was all pretty easy for me.

Preparing to have my second baby

Yeah, I think it's interesting being pregnant again now because the anxiety is more about having another child, rather than having another caesarean. And when I talk to other girls now, I very quickly try and bypass the caesarean part because you're in the hands of the professionals, and it's all going to go absolutely fine.

Whereas you're actually handing your body over to someone to operate on you. And there's a baby all of a sudden on your chest and you need to do something with it. No one else is going to do anything for you.

I think my experience actually surpassed my research. The research was quite gory. And it's quite funny; as the woman being the patient, you don't see all the blood and guts really. Unless you have a terrible experience, of course. But I didn't see any of that. It was all very positive. Hence, we're doing it again. I have been surrounded by doctors my whole life. And through the experience of going through IVF as well, a lot of blood tests, a lot of examinations. And this was actually easier than having any of that. So I would do it again in a heartbeat.

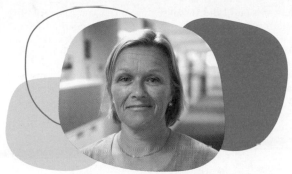

CHAPTER 7

Katie's story

I'm Katie and I had a son, Jack, when I was 35. And I had a very good pregnancy, but unfortunately, had to have an emergency caesarean section. So this is my story.

Reason for an emergency caesarean birth

At 35 weeks, I was diagnosed with preeclampsia. So I was aware that I was in and out, sort of being checked at the hospital for oedemas and protein and the blood pressure. I managed to get to full-term thanks to having medication.

Woman's experience of an emergency caesarean birth in theatre

They decided to induce me, I think it was at 40 weeks, induced me on the Sunday night. And then on the Monday, early on the Monday morning, his head hadn't … Jack's head still hadn't engaged. So it was really a question of, well okay, it's going to have to be a caesarean section. Sign here. And we'll be doing that in about 20 minutes. And then within a couple of minutes, Jack obviously went into distress. They could pick that up obviously from the monitor. And next thing I knew, I was having the epidural. I felt a bit like a rag doll. And next thing I knew, I looked up and there was my husband with the mask over his face, with his eyes looking at me. I remember this green screen lying there and there were a couple of people on the other side of it. And next thing they went, 'Here's a boy'. So it all happened very quickly.

When I was in the operating theatre itself, it wasn't an unpleasant experience. And the staff around me, including the team midwife was with me as well, were good. I didn't feel anything; it was a very strange thing to have happen to you. But overall it wasn't an unpleasant experience. And I didn't find it frightening.

The key thing for me was that Jack was healthy and I was fine.

I had felt every confidence in the obstetrician and in the midwifery team. So apart from the fact that it didn't quite end up as I'd anticipated, it was a good experience and I have a lovely son. And I can't ask for more than that and it was the best thing I ever did.

When the emergency caesarean came up, I think something that's very important is to recognise that you have every right to ask questions and be involved in the decision-making process. And I think that's very important when it comes to births.

I think it's very important that the midwives are very clear on what happens in an emergency caesarean, what you can expect to have. And at the time when you're going through that, perhaps to communicate that in a caring way but let, not too much information again, but just to keep the mother and the father aware of what's happening.

Woman's experience postnatally following an emergency caesarean birth

I was on pethidine, so I was pretty off my face, to be fairly honest. So that was a bit tricky with the breastfeeding. And in fact Nick came in one day and I was very impressed, because he literally just went, 'Look Katie, I'll deal with this for you'. And latched Jack on and away we went. So the first couple of days were … I was in a bit of a haze.

And things like the gown, I only had the gown on. It was tied up the back but of course I walked up the corridor and it was a sight for sore eyes you can imagine. So I think from a midwife's point of view, I perhaps could have had a little bit more assistance with that because I was reacting quite strongly to the pain relief. But it got better and I got used to the breastfeeding. And it was fine.

So I didn't specifically have a debrief, but the information sort of came out. And I do tend to ask questions if I'm unclear about things.

I think I liked the fact that it was the team midwifery program so I got to know the four midwives quite well. And they kept an eye on me; they told me actually when I went to leave the hospital that I was potentially vulnerable to postnatal depression, because I didn't have any family in Australia. So I appreciated that. And, yeah, overall they were very caring.

When I had the catheter removed I went to the bathroom afterwards and I didn't realise that in fact you can very often get a lot of bleeding. So I can remember pushing the panic button thinking, 'Oh my god, what's happening to me?' But everything was fine. So there are those sorts of things that they perhaps could have been a little bit clearer about the process, going through caesarean section after I'd had Jack. Just to say, 'Look, this will happen, this will happen'.

My experience with the catheter and the pethidine and the fact that you're all in a whirl with this baby, and it's just very important just to give clear guidance. Not too much information but clear guidance that's nurturing and keeping the mother on track.

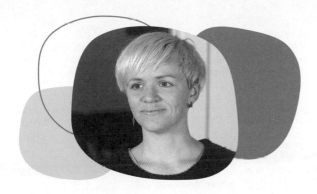

CHAPTER 8

Leia's story

My name's Leia Sidery and I'm a queer mum. And my partner Toby and I have had a little baby girl called Taj, who's 1.

Sensitive midwifery care

My friend who is also a queer parent, when dealing with health professionals, often they just assume her partner is male. And feels like when she corrects them she feels like she's being rude, by correcting them.

When a midwife gets a client who is queer or I guess they just need to keep an open mind and not judge. And ask questions, but not invasive questions that aren't necessary. So if it's about the donor sperm, just ask about the donor sperm, but you don't need to know who they are or what relationship they're going to have necessarily. Or just, I guess, test the waters before jumping in because some people are really sensitive about that kind of stuff. So, like anyone, you just need to suss out the person, I think, first before, yeah, just making any assumptions about them.

If it's just personal sort of poking around because it's something different, something new, you might want to just ask. Yeah, but it should keep things related to pregnancy and midwifery care, I think, to start with, while you're getting to know them.

I guess this applies to anyone and not just same-sex couples. Letting go of any bias you might have about them, you know, like whether it's all lesbians have short hair or whatever. And just have an open mind and, yeah, be respectful.

It would be good for student midwives to know when dealing with same-sex couples, just before you get to know them, just to suss out what they like to refer to their sperm donor as. So don't just call it 'a father' straight away; that could be offensive to some people. So just 'sperm donor' is probably the best way to start.

It's important when midwives are caring for same-sex couples just to drop any judgements that they might have, pre-conceived ideas about what queer people are like, so that they can just care for them as women.

I had continuity of care and, yes, my midwife was my mother, but just having the same woman look after you, you don't have to repeat your story to different people every time you meet someone new. You form a really close bond with them. And they care for you and I think to have that throughout a whole pregnancy is the optimal experience for a woman who's having a baby.

It shouldn't make a difference if a couple is a same-sex couple or a heterosexual couple. At the end of the day, it's people having babies, and that's the main point. And everyone should have the same care. It doesn't matter what your background is; everyone's got a different story. We're all individuals and no kind of stereotype fits anyone from any group. And I think any midwife should just care. I mean, midwife means 'with woman'. So just be with the women and care for them. That's your job.

Discriminatory behaviour

We haven't actually experienced any negativity from any health professionals, due to having a baby or being lesbian parents.

The only discriminatory issue we've had is when we moved into this house and a man started driving past our house in the middle of the night, beeping and yelling homophobic abuse at us. And I was about 8 months pregnant when it started. So he'd obviously seen us. Which is just weird to think that you'd look at two women, one who's heavily pregnant, and want to yell at them and scream abuse at them and beep your horn at them in the middle of the night. And that actually went on for about a year. And it was scary once Taj was born as well because it just felt a bit invasive and dangerous.

But I've got other friends who have experienced all kinds of horrific things from verbal, physical, sexual abuse, and not being served in shops. And people always assuming that your partner is male when you have a baby. Which is fine, 'cause people aren't meant to know. But I guess, once they do find out, not to be shocked or offended. It's okay, it's fine. It's normal for us.

Leia's story

So Toby and I, we'd actually only been together for 2 years. But, you know, when you've found the one, you know you've found the one. And we decided to have a baby. Even though I'm the younger one, I decided to go first. Well, we both decided, I think probably because of my background, mum being a midwife and all. And I was pretty excited about doing it, having a homebirth and everything.

And I always knew I wanted to have a baby and I never knew how it would actually happen, how we'd go about doing it. But I guess with anything that is 'to be', synchronicity kind of happens. My best friend's brother, Nat, one day we were out and about and I was just watching him. And it just occurred to me that he'd be the perfect father for our baby, or donor or whatever it is that he'd want to be.

So the idea kind of stuck. And the more we sort of watched him, the more we just knew. He's a performer for children. He does a lot of musical theatre kind of stuff, mainly for kids. And he's just amazing with kids. So we wrote a scroll, this beautiful scroll with like calligraphy. And we wrote like a couple of lines each to sort of ask him to sire our child. And one night, drove round to his house and dropped it in the letterbox and quickly drove away.

It took him a couple of weeks. He was like, he just burst into tears when he read the letter. But 'cause he performs and he tours a lot, he just didn't know if it was the right thing, 'cause he did want to be involved. And he always wanted to have kids but he didn't know how he'd do it either. And in the end, he took us out for dinner and said yes, that he wanted to do it.

And I think it took two tries and we got pregnant pretty much straight away. Which is good 'cause it started to get a little bit awkward after a while. It's just very, it's kind of clinical; it's not really fun like when you're doing it for months. Yeah, and the pregnancy was just awesome. It was such a beautiful experience. And having mum as my midwife, it felt very just natural and at home with it all, I guess.

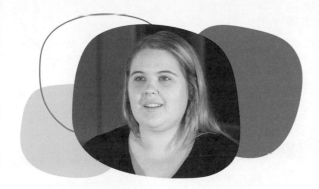

CHAPTER 9

Jordan's story

Hi, I'm Jordan. I had my first child when I was 16. The labour, I felt, went forever. I was not expecting any of it. It was all a big shock. My second child, I had when I was 19, so my daughter was 2 then, and I felt it was a lot more easy-going process. I think I enjoyed it a lot more and I knew what was going to happen.

Support for the pregnancy

So when I fell pregnant at 16, the first time I fell pregnant, it was a bit, I felt two ways about it. I think I always wanted to have children young—not that young, I don't think. But I would have always had children young. The situation for me, it's not the ideal situation for me.

And so when I fell pregnant at 16 and I decided to keep my child, my mother was very supportive. She probably didn't like the situation, as I was quite young. But she definitely respected that decision. It was more in terms of telling my dad. I think I waited until I turned 17 to tell him, 'cause I thought it sounded better. But they were very supportive, they were very supportive, so I was very lucky about that.

So being a young mum, for my antenatal care, I thought it was appropriate. I guess I didn't know anything else. I didn't know what I was supposed to … I always wanted to go to my antenatal appointments. If anything, I wanted more. I always asked questions and sometimes I felt that, in the antenatal clinic, seeing all those women, it was sort of, one in and then the next one. So I didn't feel, sometimes I felt a bit … oh you know, they don't really … I just wanted to sit there all day and talk about everything that I wanted to know. And sometimes that wasn't the case, sometimes it was. I got some really good midwives who would talk through everything. I was really excited about that. And then sometimes it was sort of straight to the point and on to next week, sort of thing. But otherwise, I enjoyed it.

For my first child, I went to antenatal classes. My mum had a friend actually, she was very lovely. She was a childbirth educator. And she was really nice. I only had a few visits; I think that's all I needed. She gave us information and she was really helpful in including my partner. I think 'cause we were really young and I think he was more immature than I was. So I think that took the stress away, of her including him and showing him sort of the things that we were going to be expecting.

Support from partner, family and friends

My partner, when I was in labour, I think he was very shocked. I have a lot of family support. So my mum was there, my aunty was there, so it's not like he was forefront expected to do everything. I think they sort of just jumped in and took lead. I don't think he really did much. I think I caught him playing on his phone at some point. I mean, in our antenatal classes, he was shown how to massage and things to expect. But I think the whole thing just completely shocked him.

So in terms of going home and caring for her, I had a lot of support. I lived at home with my parents and I think my nan and my grandpa were there at the same time as well. And my sisters, so it was all hands on deck. So I had a lot of support and I think that helped a lot. It also helped that I had a perfect baby who just slept and ate all the time. I think from 4 weeks, she slept right through the night. So I think I went back to studying, maybe a month later. So I found it really easy, yeah.

So changes after I had my daughter, was pretty much more socially. I coped really well with the baby and all things new there. But socially, things changed. Friends who I was really close with before, I wasn't too close with any more. We lost touch, obviously 'cause my priorities lied somewhere else. And I found that really difficult.

I finished Year 10. Didn't do 11 and 12, but I've been studying ever since, with both the children. I think I went back 'cause both my children were born in July. So that's when the holidays fall in any of the courses that I've done. So I've pretty much studied, had the break, had my babies and gone back straight after. I think because I've had such great babies. They've been really good. Sleep all the time, eat, perfect, so I was lucky in that regard.

Support in breastfeeding and postnatally

Postnatal, I had a few problems during my first, my first child, with breastfeeding. I felt, I think from initially in ante-natal, I decided, yep, that's what I wanted to do. I definitely wanted to breastfeed. But I didn't know anything about it. I was never given information. I assume that because I had said that's what I wanted to do.

And so afterwards, it was all sort of shocking: 'I'm so tired. I've been in labour for so long'. And my baby wanted to feed every, however many hours. And it was just so … and I just felt I'd be doing it wrong. And someone didn't come in and say, here let me help you, do this. I felt really judged. They'd come in and say, 'You're doing it wrong' or I didn't feel confident at all. And I think I was in there for a week 'cause they wanted to get the breastfeeding under way. But I was so traumatised by it that I couldn't say, at the time … I wasn't going to turn around and ask the midwife for a bottle because I didn't feel like I could. So when I went home, that's exactly what I did do. So that was really challenging, that was really hard.

Also, after I gave birth too, I was in a mothers' group, so when I went home. And they were all older. I think the youngest one, apart from me, was maybe 28. So I was really young. And I was the only one that fed my baby with formula instead of breast milk. So that was really challenging. So yeah, I had a lot of issues around breastfeeding, after that.

What could have helped postnatally, I think, perhaps being with a younger mothers' group might have helped. Sometimes I feel like I'm an exception to the rule, which is where it comes from. There's this big, what teenage mothers, how they conduct themselves and all that kind of stuff. And I feel I'm sort of the exception to the rule; I don't feel like I'm imma-ture and stuff like that. I didn't want to go to a young mothers' group initially, that's what I didn't want to do. I think they'd asked me actually and that's not something that I wanted to do. But then again, yeah, it didn't work. But I think because I had such great support at home, it wasn't a big issue for me. I didn't feel I needed it.

Midwifery care of young women

My advice for young, pregnant women to benefit from my experience is, would be to ask questions. You don't know what's going to happen, you've never been through it; it's a new experience. I know myself, teenagers think they're on top of the world. And I think just the realisation of birth and labour. And bringing up a baby and looking after a baby, what it entails. What they're actually going to be doing. I think it really needs … show pictures of labour, show videos, get them to talk to other women perhaps, anything to just … the realisation. 'Cause I think it is a big shock.

I decided to go to the birth centre for my first child, 'cause I thought, I don't need any pain relief, I'll be fine. I'm really ready for this, I'm excited, I can do it. And that was just not the case. I was so overwhelmed. I was not expecting … no one told me about prelabour; I think I prelaboured for 3 days or something. So it was just the most overwhelming experience because I just didn't know all this information that I think was really relevant. And could have maybe changed the outcome of the birth. Or even breastfeeding afterwards. So I think just information and the realisation of what's going to happen.

I just think that you shouldn't judge first off. Really need to get an understanding of who you're looking after and their support. 'Cause I just don't think my circumstances … I don't think you can throw every teenage mother into the same boat. Like I've read about where extra support and stuff like that and it's great. But I think that it needs to be tailored.

So for most of my pregnancy, for both actually, I felt that people pigeon-holed me. And sort of in a sense that I was expected to do this in a certain way. And that because I was a teenage mum, this is the things that needed to happen in order for me to have a good labour or things like that. I mean everyone's different anyway, but I think that, I felt that I was mature. And I would have liked to have been treated more as if I was, how I was feeling. Rather than what the norm is for a teenage mother.

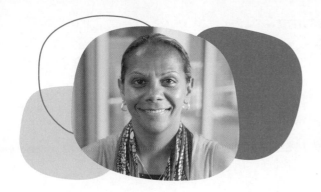

CHAPTER 10

Leona's story

My name is Leona McGrath. I am originally from Queensland. My great-grandmother's people are the Woppaburra people from Great Keppel Island. My great-grandmother was one of the last Aboriginal people taken off the island. Moved over to the mainland and then my great-grandmother moved her family down to Brisbane, on the outskirts of Brisbane. So that's where my grandmother and my mum grew up and that's where I was born.

My grandfather's people are from the Kuku Yalanji which is Far North Queensland. I grew up in Redfern, so I call Redfern, Sydney, home now.

I'm a very proud Aboriginal woman. I'm a midwife, I'm a mother to three gorgeous children and a grandmother to one beautiful little boy.

I first became interested in midwifery when I was 16 years old. I saw my sister giving birth to her first baby which was a pretty amazing experience. My mum thought it would be a good idea for me to be my sister's support person. So I was in there when she gave birth to her beautiful daughter.

Personal birth experience

I had my first daughter when I was 20 years old. I had my daughter at St Margaret's Hospital in Sydney. I had both my girls there actually. What I know now, as opposed to when I had my children, I know my experience would have been a lot different, and I think I would have had a better experience if I had another … if there was an Aboriginal midwife there. I really believe that.

I was very fortunate; I had normal births with my three children. But I do believe that my experience would have been a lot different. I had a lot of feelings of being, I suppose, a statistic. You know, we know that our Aboriginal women have their babies early and I think I felt that way, that people were sort of looking down at me and going, 'Here we go, here's another one'. Which is, you know, no woman should ever be made to feel like that regardless of her age.

But even having an Aboriginal health worker in the hospital would have made a difference, I do believe. A lot of programs that we do have across the country now that we do have Aboriginal health workers, because we do have such small numbers of Aboriginal midwives. I think that, that is helping to make things a little easier for women going into the public health system.

So my experience with pregnancy and having my children, I believe that with me having my children young and a lot of my friends and my mother speaking to me and my sister about childbirth, was that we just, you felt, pregnant is a very normal thing and we all know that as health professionals. But I think that Aboriginal women have that way of thinking, that pregnancy is normal. We do have our babies early and we just go into hospital and we have them.

Culturally appropriate maternity services

I believe my daughter's birth experience was a lot more culturally appropriate than mine as my daughter went through a service who provide care to Aboriginal women and their families. My daughter was very fortunate I think to have me as a midwife.

But also the midwives who cared for her during the antenatal period, postnatal period, and while she was having her baby, had worked with Aboriginal women before and were culturally appropriate.

The midwives who cared for my daughter understand the needs of the Aboriginal women within the communities that they work in. And they did provide appropriate care to her.

They provided appropriate care in being able to provide flexible appointments, following up with Tenisha if she didn't actually show for her appointments. They would ring her, they were able to provide care either at the hospital or at the clinic, which I think is quite important, being able to be flexible with Aboriginal women and their families, understanding the needs. I think that's why the service is so successful.

Barriers for Aboriginal women accessing antenatal care

I believe that some of the barriers for Aboriginal women accessing care is not knowing the midwives. That's why I feel that it's very important that we increase our midwifery workforce. I think the AMIHS programs in New South Wales are so successful because they do have a midwife and they have the Aboriginal health worker working alongside them, which is that connection to community.

So I think, historically, Aboriginal women view birth as a normal process. We don't feel that we need to rush in to see a doctor or a midwife as soon as we fall pregnant. We can feel our baby kicking and we've got our mums and our aunties to tell us everything's alright.

But I think that by increasing our workforce it will start changing statistics such as low birthweights, smoking in pregnancy and other chronic diseases.

Advice for midwives and midwifery students

I would advise any midwife or midwifery student looking after Aboriginal people—Aboriginal women, sorry—that if you're not sure, just ask. It's really okay to ask. I think that's one of the things that is really important that we do ask people if it's okay and if it's not okay.

Flexibility is really important when providing care to Aboriginal women and their families. Being able to provide, not being on such a tight regime when it comes to appointments and when you're offering antenatal care, and also postnatal care.

I believe another important factor that will help to change the system would be training, cultural awareness training for our staff.

I would encourage all midwifery students to complete their mandatory training, Respecting the Difference in New South Wales and whatever else other states have, as it will give you a clearer understanding of being able to communicate with Aboriginal people. And will help you in your practice when you do care for Aboriginal women and their families.

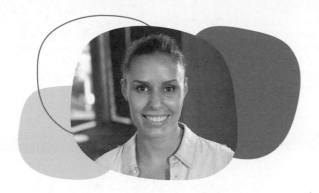

CHAPTER 10

Kate's story

Hi, my name's Kate Williams. I'm a registered nurse and a registered midwife. I'm also an Aboriginal woman. I've grown up in Sydney and my grandfather and his tribe are the Wiradjuri tribe. He was from Cowra. My dad has lived in Sydney, I've lived in Sydney in the Eastern suburbs my whole life, city urban girl. I became a registered nurse straight after school. And I became interested in midwifery and did that very soon after.

Working as a midwife

My interest in midwifery was developed sort of by chance really, initially. And that happened just through, I wanted to give back to the community. I didn't know how and I was interested in health and I thought given the huge disparities between mainstream and Aboriginal health, I thought that that would be a really good avenue to take, especially 'cause it was something I was interested in. So that started with nursing and I found it was very, the sickness model, looking after sick people. And when I came across midwifery and just jumped in, took the plunge, I found that I was looking after well people. And I really enjoyed that.

You've got a real sort of diverse day. There's a lot of autonomy. You can really build relationships with people, not just sort of seeing them come into the hospital and leave again. You can sort of see them from start to finish, which is what I got to do. And living and working in the same community, it's been really rewarding.

And the other thing that I love about midwifery is that I did always see myself wanting to make a difference in the community. And I think with so many multilayered disparities and things that can be changed, I think what better way to do it than to start with a mum and a baby and a new family and a new life. And making sure that child has the best possible antenatal care, making sure their mother's well and educated and making healthy decisions.

And by making sure that when they are born, they are getting all the appropriate checks and being referred to early childhood and getting them the referrals as necessary. And so I think by starting at that really beginning point is just a really, really effective way to make a change.

Working as a midwife in an Aboriginal maternal and infant health practice

I have worked in with the Aboriginal community. In November 2006, the Malabar Community Midwifery Links Service was established at the Royal Hospital for Women. And I had just finished my new grad rotation as a midwife, so it was perfect timing. I entered that service as in a mentored position. And we started off very small, being a new service. And the girls that I worked with were unbelievable in really sort of helping me and showing me and learning on the job really.

I got a really, really good opportunity to work with the local communities there. And we even got a lot of people coming in from interstate. It was a tertiary referral hospital, so got to have a lot of experience with that. I just absolutely … that's my passion. I absolutely love being able to provide care to my own community. I think it's unbelievable and it's really rewarding.

So the value in having a place like Malabar is it's really accessible. It's in the community. I don't know if you know logistically where La Perouse is. To go from La Perouse to the closest hospital at the Royal Hospital for Women is two buses. So if you've got two or three kids in tow, it's raining, you'd have got a lot of other priorities, going to an antenatal appointment is really not high on the list of priorities. Especially being a really culturally appropriate, accessible place, we found that the women were actually presenting earlier. We were getting some really good results and some good feedback and slowly we became busier and busier because the community just learned to trust you and understand that you're there and become a lot more comfortable with you. And we found that not only was it really sort of job satisfaction for us, it was really, the results were speaking for themselves.

The Malabar service is very different to the other services in the hospital because it was a caseload practice. So there was a group of four midwives. And we provided the antenatal care, intrapartum care and postnatal care at home. We would come up to the ward and visit the women day 1, day 2 or even day 3 sometimes on the ward. And it was very flexible. The women often found it very difficult to say, 'Well, how many visits do I get?' 'Well, how long do I stay in the hospital?' And it took a while for people to understand well, it's completely flexible.

You can come and stay for as long as you need and when you're happy to go home, within a reasonable timeframe, between sort of 24 and 72 hours, we'll come and visit you whenever you need. We're on the end of the phone, you can call us anytime. And if you need a visit, we'll be there. And if you're fine, we won't be. And it was just that you found that the women, even though they thought they would want a lot of visits, it actually instilled a lot of confidence. That they actually would go home and maybe not call you as much as you thought they would or they thought they would. It had a really good effect on the women and I think they really appreciated to know that if they needed us, we would be there.

It was a very flexible service because, it's quite hard to understand because it is so flexible. We often did antenatal appointments at the Aboriginal Medical Service at Redfern. We would do home antenatal appointments if the woman couldn't make the facility. We would often go down to La Perouse to the Aboriginal Health Service down there. In terms of their birthing, yes it was at the Royal Women's.

The midwives would carry around, we would carry around a phone and whoever was on call would, that phone was on. And it would ring at any time. The women in labour, ruptured membranes, any reason that they called they could call. And if it was time to come in and have their baby, if they were in labour, they would come in and we would follow them in and meet them there. So they had the opportunity to go to the birth centre, they could go to delivery suite or, if there were any complications and ended up transferred to theatre for a caesarean, we would also follow the women through for that. So it really was a continuity of care model.

Reflections on specific cultural practices

So specific cultural practices, I don't think I've had a great deal of that, specifically being in such an urban area. The only thing I can say from my perspective is that the hospital system is usually quite rigid and has rules and two people per room or something like that. And you'll find with the Aboriginal community, it's really normal to have really large numbers of family or close people in their lives, in the birth.

So I've been at births where there's been 15 people in the room. And I know a lot of people would find that really off-putting. At certain times you could find that people were being a bit distracting, but usually it was just really normal. I don't know how else to describe it. And the birthing process a lot of the times is just really normal. People expect there that it's going to hurt, or they've got aunties or grandmothers or friends who have all birthed as well, who sort of give them advice. They just get on with it. They just do it, a lot of the time. So it's great to be a part of.

Postnatally, some of the things that I've seen myself, that I've observed, is that you will get a lot more co-sleeping with a lot of the Aboriginal community. We just talk about education, about the safety of that. And providing that it's done really safe, which it really is. You'll find that that's a lot more evident. The breastfeeding rates are pretty good.

I think the most important thing when caring for an Aboriginal or Torres Strait Islander person is to ask. Don't be afraid to ask are you Aboriginal or Torres Strait Islander? Sometimes people are a bit, sort of put off about asking that in case it's offensive but it really isn't. And the culture is very, very different. And by asking that question, you can maybe offer specific services, culturally appropriate services. In which case that might have an impact on that woman's journey.

I would also not just group all Aboriginal people together in one basket. Everyone's different and that's the same for the Aboriginal community as well. And if you're not sure of something, just ask. It's a really nice thing, I think, for anyone, not just Aboriginal people, to ask, you know, how are you going, did you understand that? And just explaining what you're doing. Don't just tell people, 'This is what we're doing'.

It's just really nice to sort of explain things, have a conversation. Maybe not try and be too time pressured. I know that's really difficult to say with the time pressures that you have. I can understand that better than anyone. But if you just take that time to sit down and have a conversation and really engage and make sure the person's understood what you're saying, I think that's a really good practice and I think that's good practice all round really.

Sometimes when working with the Aboriginal community, you just need to be aware that things don't fit into nice, neat, little boxes all the time. Especially when you're out in the community. Sometimes you do need to be a little bit flexible. And just do things a little bit differently sometimes to get a really good result. Definitely stay within your scope of practice and definitely work within safety guidelines and everything.

Reflections on working for the NSW Ministry of Health

I've been at the Ministry now for just over a year. I've been seconded there for 2 years. I was in the Royal Hospital for Women in the Malabar Service for 6½ years and I was on call. And I absolutely loved it and that's my absolute passion working clinically with the community. But I just found that I really needed a break from that. And so rather than moving away or getting out of midwifery completely, I thought I would just have a look at my options and this job came up in the Aboriginal Nursing and Midwifery Strategy.

So, although I get to help the community in a very different way now, it's certainly broadened my horizons and taught me a lot. I've never sort of not worked clinically before which has been really eye-opening. And it's been great because you can actually help the community in other ways.

So we're looking at things like recruitment and retention of Aboriginal nurses and midwives in the system. We're looking at rewriting a new strategy. We do scholarships and cadetship programs to help support Aboriginal people to increase the numbers in the New South Wales public health system in the workforce. We know that to have a culturally competent workforce, not only does mainstream staff need to be culturally aware, but it's great to have a few black faces around, to be honest. It's really nice to walk somewhere and see you have that connection and I think it makes a real difference.

Aboriginal people have historically not wanted to access mainstream services. It's just part of our history. And so by changing that, by changing the culture of the workplace, by being more aware, I think people will be much more likely to access those services and, in turn, improve their health outcomes, of themselves and their families.

So I think that with more and more services like Malabar, AMIHS services, community-based services, and by having more Aboriginal people within these services to help and encourage people and educate people along the way, I think that rather than having these small, little groups of them everywhere, by really integrating it into the system, I think it's going to make a huge difference. And I certainly hope it does.

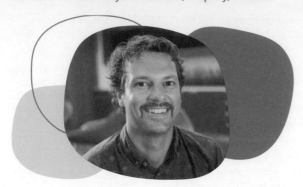

CHAPTER 11

Simon's story

My name's Simon Smith. I am a father of three kids, who were all born at home. I live on the mid-north coast of New South Wales in Sawtell. I'm a music teacher and I go for the Rabbitohs.

Preparing for birth and fatherhood

I felt like I was prepared, and I felt like I really knew the midwives because Jac had a homebirth and there was a lot of visits. And the midwives would come to our house and I got to ask a lot of questions. I got to know them more personally. I got to understand their characteristics and I got to build a sense of trust between myself and Jane, our midwife, and Ali.

And when the pregnancy came to the birthing part of it, I guess, the labour, their personalities, I knew I could trust them. I felt safe with them, but the whole energy changed because it was this sacred birthing space that I wasn't aware that would happen. Which happened to be our kitchen, in Newtown, for our first child being born.

And, yeah, I just had lots of jobs to do and I don't think I was 100% prepared, but I don't know if anyone is ever 100% prepared for watching their first child being born right there and then. And as for fatherhood, that's an ongoing thing and I don't know if I ever will be either. We got a fridge magnet when Eva was born. It said, 'The first 40 years are always the hardest' and I think they might be right.

Engaging with the midwives

The type of jobs that I had to do, I found out in the meetings leading up to the birth. So the midwives would come to our house and visit Jac and see how she was going and bring the Doppler and check the baby. And I got to be part of that whole process, which I think helped prepare me for the birth. And in that time, they told me the roles that they were going to take on.

So Nicky took on a role of sitting back and observing and making sure everything was going. And she would take notes and wrote beautiful little anecdotes and quotes of what was being said to one another. And jotted the time down as significant events occurred. And Ali took on a role of like working the hot towels and bringing things and taking photographs. Nicky also had the video camera, that was her sort of role.

And then Jane, I guess you would have said, was the primary midwife. And she was basically right in close with Jac most of the time. And Ali and her would sort of tag in, tag out, which gave me the role of getting everything together firstly, which I loved doing, getting a checklist, feeling like I had a role of getting the birth pool, getting the pasta scoop to scoop the stuff out of the birth pool.

And figuring out how the birth pool works, filling it up, testing it out, watching the cricket lying in it. And then figuring out where to drain it, how to drain it, connecting the taps. Doing all sorts of manly stuff that I don't normally do 'cause that's not my thing, but yeah, it made me feel important, so that was good.

And it also made me feel a lot safer knowing that I was okay to be supporting Jac because the midwives around me, I knew what they were doing and I knew that I didn't need to be Superman doing everything because it was a homebirth. And I really felt like my role was clearly there to support my partner.

Experience of becoming a father

First time of being a father was intense, I guess. I always make a strange noise when every one of my children are born and the first time was no different. I make a sort of sound that Harold Bishop, I think from *Neighbours*, makes, a 'huuh' sort of sound. It was a magical time. She was born in our kitchen and all the midwives did amazing things while we took our beautiful baby girl into our lounge room.

And, yeah, sleeplessness. Trying to figure out what my role is, how much I should do, how much I could do, that was the hardest thing for me. I wanted to be supportive, but I took it too far in the sense that I was useless because I hadn't rested at all. So it was no point in me trying to help too much, so that took the mother-in-law to say, 'Simon, snap out of it, you can't do everything. Have a sleep. Figure out what you can do and then you'll be of more use to us'. Which was tough love, but valid. A valid point.

I guess being someone who was very independent and did whatever I wanted before a child, like before a child came into our lives, I think a negative thing was figuring out that life's not just about me anymore. I need to share my life with my child. Like, in saying that, I shared it with my wife, but we, I don't know, it just went without saying we've been together that long, we obviously share it together.

But, yeah, having this entity that was totally dependent, needed to be carried. And Eva needed to be put to sleep in a pram sitting up. And then when she went to sleep you'd have to slowly lie it back down and then wheel it into the front room. And she was so spoilt, it was ridiculous. So yeah, the third one didn't get any of this treatment. But anyway, so just balancing time for myself, for my wife and for our child, that was a hard thing to figure out at the start, I guess, as a negative.

The most stressful part about becoming a father, I guess, is keeping them alive, my children. The visits to hospital when they fall off their bikes or out of trees or bikes fall out of trees and hit them in the head as has happened to my youngest one a couple of weeks ago, so usual stuff like that. So kids getting sick, I guess that's been the most stressful part of it. And I guess and the work, life, family balance. I guess that's the stressful part. And just time, being time poor, sharing that limited finite thing that is time, between one another.

Engaging fathers

The importance of engaging fathers, I guess. Firstly I'd like to say about engaging fathers, I think birth is secret women's business. And I think that it's amazing what happens in that birthing space. I think the benefit of engaging a father is the connection I get with my child when I'm part of that. And the way the midwives that helped me do that was basically give me things that I could do. And give me active jobs, like I said earlier.

So giving me a list of things to prepare. So preparing the birth kit, so whether you're having your child at home or at a hospital, preparing, giving that job to the dad or the partner, to prepare that so they feel connected to the pregnancy and the baby that's going to be born, so that there's an active role to be played.

Consciously saying that your role is just to be supportive of your partner—that was a really great thing for me to hear that I didn't need to do everything. I needed just to be supportive. And actually hear it, it sounds like a given. But just to hear that from our midwives was a really great thing for me and I found really helped me focus on my wife and her while she was having our babies.

The other thing that helped me connect to the whole birthing process was, I was taken to the room where, say if a vacuum had to happen and stuff, and I was actually shown some of the equipment that would be used, so it didn't seem so foreign. It thankfully didn't have to happen, but just knowing what a room looks like

So I went into St George Hospital and I went into a room where you might have to use this equipment and this is what this is for. And so obviously midwives don't always have that much time to do such things, but it was really nice to see that equipment. So I could imagine it would be really stressful for a partner to see these things for the first time in an emergency situation where these are required. So to see this stuff not just in a book and stuff, yeah, that helped me as well.

Ways that midwives could recommend to get dads closer to their babies is, I guess, incorporating them in the process of the pregnancy, like coming to the meetings that they go to before the baby's born. I don't know the technical names of all these things, sorry. And involving them in the birth process and then afterwards just connections. Things like holding the baby, using things like Hug-a-Bubs, which are impossible to tie up, but once you figure them out, they're great. Like, I remember putting my daughter inside ours and putting a jacket around it and sneaking in to the members' section to watch the Swannies play because you're not allowed to take kids in there. Stuff like that. That was a really nice way that I bonded with my daughter.

Other ways, just walking with a pram around the block. Carrying her in the night sometimes when Jac was sick of breastfeeding and needed sleep. And handing her to me and just standing there walking around the table numerous times while she fell asleep. And then sitting down and her waking up and crying again and doing it again. All those things, they were horrible at the time and I thought they'd last forever, but I don't know, they helped build that bond between myself and my child.

Bathing the baby, I did mostly in the shower. So for ways to bond with the child, we didn't really do the bathing with Eva because she hated it. She hated going in the bath but Jac would hand her to me in the shower, which was a really nice thing to do.

I was really paranoid about dropping her because my brother-in-law had had a slippery incident where that had occurred. So, yeah, got to be careful, but that's a good way too, in the shower. That was really good. As for the baby massage, we got the book and stuff but I just never got around to reading it. I think I was too tired.

I found the books that the midwives recommended to me from the birth centre at St George. *New Active Birth* was a book that I read that I remember and *Baby Watchers*, I can't remember who that's by, and there's one other book that escapes me, I'll find it out and let you know as soon as possible which one that was. But, the books were great. I read them a lot during the first pregnancy and they really helped prepare me, I guess, for the physiological things that were going to happen to Jac. Not so much the psychological.

My midwives and my wife helped inform me enough to know that this is a rite of passage of life that should be celebrated, not feared. So I guess, yeah, they were the negative things that I'd hear most and I still do when I tell people about my kids' birth experiences. And I hear their stories. It generally comes from a place of fear and that fear, I think, is from not being fully informed and aware of what's going on, I guess.

The thing I would like to see new midwives doing for fathers is including them in the process, helping them find places where they can become informed, and encouraging them to ask questions and feel safe in the space because they know how important that space is, I guess. That would be the main thing I would ask new midwives to do, if they could.

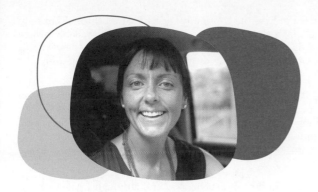

CHAPTER 12

Cassandre's story

Hi, I'm Cass. I'm mum of four children; two sets of twins. There's Samuel and Thomas that are 4 and Scarlett and Jacob that are almost 10 months.

Decision making regarding mode of birth

I was happy with the end result. We were all fit and well and healthy, but it was just the process of getting there when I look back. Didn't really have that consistency of care. When I turned up to the high-risk clinic each week, I was seen by a different registrar. And although it was documented in the medical notes, the plan of care and what the next action was, that particular registrar had maybe a different viewpoint. And, 'Oh, no, no, we don't need to do that', or … from early on, I was looking for a planned C-section just purely speaking with friends that were within the medical career.

And I suppose as well looking at that, I was away from home and just felt maybe my personal background, it could give me the security there to know that we were all healthy. And the position of the babies towards the end led me to believe that that would be the right decision to take for a planned C-section. But I really had to fight my way to get there, to be honest. And it wasn't until I requested to see the consultant, Dr Davison, he told me on appointment, 'Well, your first baby would come out fine, but I really wouldn't be concerned. We most probably would have to take you through for a C-section after'.

And it was that that made me think, well I don't actually want to go through two experiences in one day really. If you were thinking I could hopefully give birth naturally to two, I would give it a whirl, but when you're already thinking that most probably would have to have a C-section then, yes I was more than happy just to plan for that.

Yeah, looking back, in retrospect, I s'pose at the time I did wonder to myself would I regret that I really did push for a planned C-section. But initially and still now, I'm so glad I did, to be honest. The second twin, Thomas, he was actually wedged up in my rib cage and they did have difficulty getting him out and it turned out to be that his birthweight was three percentiles lower than what he had been on all my scans that I had through my pregnancy. He was fine but just for the parameters of weight, he was below average and had to be in special care for two nights.

So I just wonder if I had gone for the natural, whether things may have been different, but I mean, you don't know. But I was more than happy, we were all healthy and that's just really what I wanted was two healthy babies and a healthy mummy.

The course of the pregnancies/births

So both pregnancies were natural. And a very big surprise the first time round, never mind the second time round, to find out that I was pregnant with twins. The nausea started first time round from 7 weeks and carried on pretty much up until … sounds very bizarre and I know people laugh at me now, the nausea lifted soon as I had the C-section and was on that operating table. I just instantly could feel like it had gone, bizarrely.

And same with the second time round with the babies, but it was a lot harder second time round with having two infants round my ankles to have to entertain. And couldn't quite just put myself to bed every day and had to just try and prioritise and rest as and when I could, in between entertaining the boys, bless them.

Both sets of twins went full-term, 38 plus 4, if I'm right in saying. So the birth itself was really, I suppose, as I expected. I was very anxious in the way of having a spinal block, but the theatre team, the anaesthetist, they were just wonderful, very, very supportive. Yeah, explained everything and I think that was just really what I needed. I can recall actually a theatre nurse had just come over when the anaesthetist was just setting up. And said, 'I think you could maybe do with a cuddle. Would you mind?' And she asked permission, but it was just, I've never had anybody be so open and out there with a cuddle before. But do you know, actually, it was just what I needed and it just got me in that next frame of mind to, 'Right this is it, we're gonna have the babies'.

So second time round I saw the clinical midwife consultant all the way through. So I think that really gave me a different journey, more of a positive journey.

So in the way of your medical care, would be ideally pushed for to have the continuity there. 'Cause I think if I'm right in saying how it still is at the moment, with the high-risk clinic, is that you do just see the GP that's available, which just really—sorry, the registrar that's available at the clinic at that time—which I s'pose in one respect, the positive side of it could be that you're getting a different set of eyes looking into your case each week, so you're getting a broader spectrum.

But where you're not getting that continuity there which, I feel that I personally really did need, and I think every mum-to-be and family-to-be does need, so yeah, try and push to have somebody there to follow you through your journey pathway. Whether it is a registrar that would be willing to see your case through, or maybe a midwife that could see you at high-risk clinic each time. But somebody there to follow you through and help you along your journey.

Postnatal care

In the way of the aftercare, when I look back, I did really have two different experiences. And although I had both sets of twins at Wollongong Hospital, I don't know, looking back now, if it was a mixture of things—that an English young lady that had just immigrated, no support network. My viewpoint, I just wonder if some professional sort of categorised and just saw all these alarm bells ringing. And I could see, yes, where they were maybe coming from, but I just wonder if they just didn't quite project that in the right way.

From word go I was felt, to feel that I didn't know what I was doing. And one of the babies was taken off to special care and no explanation was given from that point. It was just protocol from what they were telling me. And we will have to give him formula, where I didn't see he needed formula, 'cause I'd not even been given the opportunity to try and feed him.

Yeah and the first couple of nights it was quite hard really to get a midwife to bring Tom to me so I could feed him. I'd had a C-section so I couldn't, and I was busy with Sam, couldn't get to special care to feed him and just felt I was a burden in one respect. But I was maybe putting myself under more pressure. 'Why would you do this? He's in special care. Let's just give him formula and you've got enough to be worrying about than to be worrying about feeding him.' And it just really contradicted what I thought the ethos of midwives was and particularly in those early stages, should be about the breastfeeding and supporting mums through that journey. But there was the other extreme of, I think it was my third night in, a different midwife, and she was just wonderful, bless her. And yeah, couldn't have helped me enough.

So when I look back, this particular midwife, how she made me feel and how she really changed my whole journey round for me, was I think she just stepped back and listened to me and listened to what I felt I wanted and needed. And what was important to me at that time and what I felt was important to me and my babies. And she listened to the fact that I actually needed a loved one around 'cause I had two babies and I was in a room on my own.

And from word go, I'd requested for my partner to stay but was told it wasn't policy. But yeah, third night, she was on and she rang James and he could come in and he could stay. And she assisted with the feeding and got me in the position that I wanted to be in and not what the midwife felt was looked like the correct position. Yes, and straight away, feeding was as it was during the days when my mum and my partner were there and a midwife wasn't there.

But I was just allowed to do what I felt comfortable and felt was best for myself and the babies. And looking back to my last experience being in the hospital, completely different journey. But I think for the sake that I don't know if because I'd already given birth to a set of twins, that people, midwives, looked upon it as, 'Well, she knows what she's doing'. I don't know, I just had a completely different journey. Was asked at all times what I felt I needed. Did I need help with attachment? Did I need anything? They were more in the background and made aware that they were available if I need them, rather than in the frontline and 'it must be done this way' and 'it must be done that way'. More of a supportive role model than an authoritative, 'this is how it should be done' role model.

The importance of family and routines

My family pretty much tag-teamed. So the children, Sam and Tom, was allowed in and the midwives were wonderful in the way that, even through rest time, but it just worked well for Sam and Tom to come in. That they could just pop in for 10 minutes and see mum and the babies.

They were more than happy to let my family tag-team to help with me and the babies. And I think that was the big thing this time round was, yes there was the hospital policy and that this is rest hour and this is not visiting hour, but as long as we were being right for the other patients and not being too noisy, which I could completely understand. We were tucked away in a room away from everybody. They were allowed to come and go really, as they pleased.

Thinking of the breastfeeding and I s'pose really my big thing, what worked with the boys and what works with Scarlett and Jacob this time round, is routine. I know when I speak to friends and other mums that are breastfeeding, a lot that

I know anyway, seem to, they feed on demand and very much into the demand feeding. Which is wonderful, it works for them. But I did try it with Sam and Tom. So my first set of twins for the first maybe 10 days, I sort of pushed it out to. But I think I would have gone a little bit crazy and definitely wouldn't still be breastfeeding.

So now my support at home is there's myself and the four children. I've got a wonderful mum that's currently over here on a tourist visa that we're just in the midst of disputing and things. But yes, thank goodness to my mum, bless her.

Got my partner as well, but he, like many households, is the main breadwinner. And he's at work 6 days a week. Works in Sydney, so he's got the commute there. So generally we're all still in bed as he leaves and all the children are back in bed as he comes home. So, yes, I don't know where I would be if it wasn't for my mum, bless her. She keeps the house afloat and everyone ticking happily, bless her.

I suppose the only real thing I come here thinking was, for me, has been routine. Because you speak to any other parent, and I know me and James will laugh and we're like, 'These parents with just single children, just do whatever'. And I suppose we have had, we've got 'twin friends' that do whatever, but bless them, they're barking crazy mad. And it's been for us, it's been … routine works and keeps us all sane. It means we can function again the next day again and be happy and blossom.

Being labelled as 'high risk'

Yeah, I s'pose looking back, the name itself, a high-risk clinic, that I felt as though you're categorised high risk, all these endless possibilities could happen. And I know going to the clinic each week and you could be sat waiting for a period of time. Speaking to the other mums to be, yeah, quite anxious of they could go into premature labour and this could happen and that could happen. And I suppose maybe for me what worked was not to necessarily take all that on board and just to listen to me, myself and my body and go with how I felt. Rest as and when I could. Which I think I've already said was harder the second time round but I did still do that.

I s'pose how I balanced that was second time round, I just made a point of really eating well and keeping up my intake that way. But yeah, I s'pose really was to block out all the negativity there of the 'high risk' and 'all these things could happen'. Because yes, they could happen but at the same time, there's no guarantee that it's gonna happen. And I just wonder, for me, to get on that spiral of negative thinking and this could happen, that could happen, that I could be a bit of a whittler anyway. So it wasn't worth going down that 'let's worry about it' pathway. We're gonna just take each day as it comes and speak up when I need to and that was what worked with that.

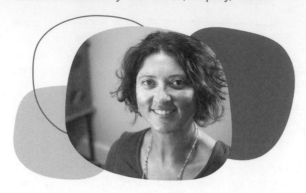

CHAPTER 13

Kathryn's story

My name's Kathy and I work as a Clinical Nurse Consultant in perinatal and infant mental health.

Overview of perinatal mental health disorders

So just to start with, I just want to make the comment that perinatal mental health issues can occur anywhere from conception up to 1 year after baby is born. Anxiety and depression are some of the most common perinatal mental health issues women may face. Anxiety could occur on its own and depression could occur on its own. Or women may experience symptoms of both. The symptoms are always on a continuum, so some women may experience the symptoms in a mild to moderate form. Others may experience these disorders in a more severe form, meaning that it affects their day-to-day functioning and also their relationship with the baby.

There is a small number of women, so probably 1 or 2 per 1000, that might experience a postnatal psychosis. So those women may—it's quite a rapid onset—so those women might start to become quite confused very quickly and also lose touch with reality. And that obviously needs quite urgent attention.

So for women with pre-existing mental health issues, such as schizophrenia and bipolar disorder, the perinatal period is a time when they're more vulnerable to relapse.

There's a range of risks that have been identified that place some women at risk of perinatal mental health issues. And I guess the more risks identified, then the greater the vulnerability for that woman, for developing perinatal mental health issues. So factors like a previous history of anxiety, depression or another mental illness. There might be psycho-social factors such as lack of support, financial issues, housing issues, domestic violence.

There's also women who have experienced childhood abuse and trauma. So for those women, becoming pregnant might reactivate memories and feelings of their own experiences of being parented. So often then they will start to think about, 'Will I be a good enough parent?', 'Will I know how to be a parent?' And often these kind of thoughts will cause them to start feeling anxious and depressed.

So the signs and symptoms of perinatal mental health issues I guess will depend on the particular issue that the woman is presenting with. If we think about anxiety, anxiety can manifest in a number of different ways. So a woman may experience generalised type anxiety, so worrying excessively about a particular issue. So in the perinatal context that might be worrying about the birthing experience, for example.

For some, anxiety might manifest as panic attacks. So these are kind of sudden, unpredictable attacks of anxiety that manifest physically. So women might experience a sudden onset of shortness of breath, feeling sweaty, trembly and they might start to have thoughts that they're losing control or they're going mad. Other women might experience unpleasant or intrusive thoughts that they feel they can't control. And then to alleviate those intrusive thoughts, they might engage in behaviours, like ritual behaviours, such as hand-washing, to alleviate that.

Depression, there's a number of symptoms that people might identify if they become depressed. There'll be changes in sleep and appetite, feeling teary a lot of the time for no good reason, feeling a lack of energy, lack of motivation, lack of confidence, feelings of hopelessness and helplessness. And I guess, at worst, feeling like they don't want to be here any more.

Symptoms, midwifery care and resources available

The symptoms might go unrecognised 'cause they can develop slowly over time. And sometimes the women themselves, or the people around them, might describe them as being hormonal or the normal ups and downs of pregnancy. So people will let symptoms go. Often on the outside, the woman might appear to be functioning quite normally, and so they go unrecognised.

I think often if people are experiencing the symptoms, they might feel a lot of shame. So to say that they're not enjoying their pregnancy or, in the postnatal period, they're not enjoying their baby, they're feeling motherhood's difficult, might be hard for them to say to the people around them. And so people tend to hide their symptoms.

So from a clinician point of view, sometimes we can be quite busy with the task that we need to attend to. So, for example, in an antenatal setting, there's very physical checks we need to attend to. There's time constraints, so there may not be space to ask the woman about how she's feeling. So, if she's not given that space, perhaps, she might not disclose really what's happening for her. I think there's a number of reasons why, perhaps, they can go unrecognised.

Midwives can provide information to women about the signs and symptoms of perinatal mental health issues, and who they can approach, should they identify these issues in themselves. So midwives can talk to women about, not only how to take care of themselves physically during pregnancy, but also emotionally. And I think the psychosocial screening at the first antenatal visit is vital for identifying risk factors. And through that process, midwives can have a role in directing women to the appropriate resources or services to support them in minimising those risk factors.

I also think midwives can have a role in identifying protective factors and strengths through that screening process. So, for example, if a woman has been depressed before and seen a psychologist, then it's likely that she has some understanding of the symptoms of depression and is likely to be able to identify them again, should they occur. And also have some understanding of what support's helped her in the past, so she can draw from that experience in the future.

I think there's a number of resources that women could access in the community, if they were to become concerned that they were developing a mental health issue in the perinatal period. Firstly, obviously the midwife, then there's the local general practitioner. I think it's really important that women make connections with their local child and family nurse as well, who could also be a good resource, in terms of letting them know who they could see in the community that might be able to assist them. Different states may offer specific perinatal and infant mental health services and women could access those resources as well.

Midwives can help by asking a woman about how she's feeling and making it part of routine care. The midwife can also be a resource for the woman, in terms of being able to give her information about where she can access appropriate resources to support her, with whatever the particular issue is. And the midwife can also be that consistent, reliable person that the woman can turn to during the pregnancy, and feel that she can talk to about any potential issues that arise.

And I do actually think that sometimes that relationship can be enough, depending on the particular issue, to support that woman through the pregnancy. So, for example, if it's very much anxiety, say for example, around the birthing process, then I think the midwife can actually hold that woman throughout the pregnancy and manage that anxiety, in that relationship.

Treatment

The course of treatment for perinatal mood disorders will vary according to the severity of the symptoms and also how those symptoms are impacting on the woman's level of functioning. And also the relationship with her baby. So for some women, they may need to increase their social networks and they might need some practical support.

Other women may need counselling around how to manage the symptoms that they're experiencing. But also counselling around the factors that might be contributing to the feelings they're having. Some women may need medication, such as antidepressants. And for some women they may need a combination of all these treatments.

Importance of treatment

It's really important for babies to have consistent, reliable and responsive caregivers. And this helps them to form a secure attachment. And we know that for babies, a secure attachment helps lay a foundation for good social and emotional development across the lifespan. If mum is depressed, it could manifest in a number of different ways in terms of the impact on the relationship with her baby.

So she might become quite withdrawn from the baby, feel resentful towards the baby. On the other side, she may become very vigilant about the baby's welfare and become quite intrusive in her parenting style. So those interactions will affect that developing attachment relationship and, therefore, potentially impact on that baby's social and emotional development.

In terms of partners, partners can also be at increased risk of developing depression if the primary caregiver is depressed. Their workload might increase, because they're not only caring for their partner, but also perhaps taking on some of the responsibilities of the baby. And also, perhaps engaged in paid work as well, so their workload is going to increase. I think partners can also feel quite helpless and hopeless, and not know what to do.

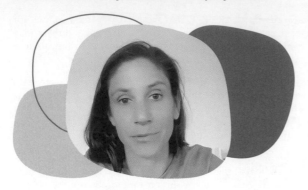

CHAPTER 13

Amy's story

My name is Amy Hannaford, I am 39 years old. I'm married to Nick, who is also 39, and together, we have four children. We have Laura, who is 13; Dylan, who is 10; Freya, who is eight; and Kira, who's six.

Different pregnancy experiences

My last pregnancy was with Kira. That one, I was okay, it was pretty good. My third pregnancy was a bit more complicated. And during the pregnancy, I got quite unwell with various viruses, I guess from having two young children who passed on a few bugs. And I think, at the time, we were living in Western Australia in Perth, and my husband Nick was working in a job that involved flying in and out of a remote area of Western Australia, off the coast of Western Australia. So, I was quite exhausted, actually, a lot. And during the pregnancy, I had an ongoing cough from the virus that I had. And I was trying to manage two children, one of whom was doing all sorts of sports at quite a young age, probably too much, excessively so, I think, for a preschooler/kindergartener. And I was just trying to really sort of get by at a high level while being pregnant and having a husband away and no family over there as well. So, it was a tough pregnancy, probably also because of, you know, my circumstances, I guess. And, yeah, I think I was exhausted when I ended up giving birth to Freya in October of 2013.

Reflecting on pregnancy and birth

I've always been a person who has tried to cope, I guess, and I guess have things 'done well'. I'm a perfectionist. I don't like making mistakes. I like to be decisive and make good decisions about everything. My previous two pregnancies (before Freya), my second child in particular, was fairly fast. And probably out of concern that I would not make the hospital, I opted to go into a home birth program, which was run through King Edward Memorial Hospital in Perth. And I felt that was a really good option because it meant that I would have someone, a caregiver, at home with me when I had Freya, and I didn't have to worry about the fact that we didn't really have family here and we weren't rushing around, and I didn't end up giving birth in a car or on the side of the road or something. So, I was quite worried and anxious about that, which was the basis for my decision to have a home birth.

Valuing evidence-based care and feeling safe

I'm someone who's quite medically minded, and I'm fully vaccinated. My children are vaccinated, and I did find that there was a level of sentiment among some of the midwives that I saw during my pregnancy where they questioned vaccination, and I had to organise the vaccines for my newborn. They didn't do that. We had some issues just before I gave birth. I tested positive for Group B strep. And at the birth, the midwife didn't bring any antibiotics, because they don't normally. And so, I was a bit stressed about that. And so, I guess there were some alternate views I didn't expect from caregivers. I did have a level of worry during the pregnancy and at birth. And so, what had been important to me, which was a home birth that, I guess, provided some sense of security around making sure everyone was safe. There were some moments when I felt unsafe, but the birth was actually great. I didn't have any issues, and Freya didn't have any issues relating to Group B strep, so that wasn't a problem. She didn't need antibiotics afterwards, I monitored her temperature, and all was well. The difficulties I had after were that everyone packed up and left, probably from feeling a bit worried at the birth, we started Freya's life with, I guess, was like an explosion. I'll never have a home birth again. What was important to me during the birth (was) just to make sure that everyone was safe and that I was safe. I feel, though, maybe I didn't feel safe for parts of it.

Having an unsettled baby and feeling isolated

Freya was born, and she just cried a lot, all the time. I barely slept for the first year of her life. In the first 12 weeks, I sought help from my GP. I remember sort of standing in my GP's room, sort of pleading with her, I kept saying, 'Something's wrong with this baby. I don't know what's wrong with her.' And the GP didn't know what to do, either. So, they referred Freya to a paediatrician. The paediatrician took bloods and ultimately came to the conclusion that Freya was just a baby that didn't want to be in a baby's body, and she appeared to be quite frustrated. But it didn't help the situation because I still had a baby that never slept and cried all the time and didn't want to be held by anyone other than me. And so that was tough. I had two other children to look after as well, and we were living in Western Australia with no family and, you know, two young children to look after and get to school, and I couldn't drive anywhere because Freya used to scream in the car a lot. And then I just wasn't sure where to turn, you know. I didn't know whom to turn to for help. So that caused a lot of difficulties, especially for someone who's always had everything organised and under control.

Relationships and bonding

It was tough. My husband and I struggled to bond with Freya because she was very difficult. There weren't moments that we enjoyed, I think, with her. I remember trying to get out to go for walks without her and leaving her with my husband. He'd just call me and ask me to come home because she just screamed and screamed and screamed. I remember him saying things like, 'I just want to throw her out the window because she just won't stop crying.' And I remember feeling that way, too. She was so difficult, I couldn't settle her at all. She was really hard work, and I think that then affected, you know, our relationship with the other two children because our time was taken up looking after Freya a lot. And so, you know, I don't actually remember much of my son's toddlerhood because it was just all taken up with caring for this baby that cried a lot. So that was really hard. I think it affected our relationship, our marriage. We went to counselling, you know, probably more just to try and feel better about everything because it's really hard. I think back on that period now and just wonder how we got through it because it was just so tough. It's so strange that a small person can have that impact on your life. Anyway, she's lovely. She's such a lovely kid, and she crawled very, very early. I think she crawled at about three months. And then she was walking at seven months and talked before 12 months. So, she really probably was just a baby that didn't like being in a baby's body.

A cry for help – treatment and support

After 12 weeks, I think she was about three months old, I went to my GP and said, 'Look, I'm not coping at all. I'm not getting any sleep, and I think I'm depressed. I don't know.' And so, my GP prescribed an antidepressant. I've never taken an antidepressant before, and she gave me a script for some Lorazepam to address any side effects of the antidepressant. And then I had quite a serious reaction to the antidepressant. So that caused quite a major turn of events because I went from sort of feeling pretty crappy, and very, very tired, to having thoughts of self-harm. And that was really eye-opening and quite traumatic. One evening I sent a message to a friend and said, 'Look, I can't cope with this any more. I just can't. I'm not sleeping. I'm done.' And I took quite a large dose of Lorazepam, and I woke up in a hospital room with heart monitors. A friend, who was in England, had taken various steps to get someone to break into our house and called an ambulance.

From there I had to book into a mother-and-baby unit. I did that as a voluntary patient. Fortunately, we have a mother-and-baby unit in Western Australia, in Perth. I was able, fortunately, to get a bed there with Freya. And I spent two months there trying to find a medication that worked, which was also very difficult. So that was tough. In the mother-and-baby unit, we had Mothercraft nurses who spent a lot of time with Freya, trying to help her learn how to self soothe, which didn't really work. But we did manage to do things like get her to take a dummy, and she accepted a bottle so I could have a break from time to time and someone else could feed her. And over that period, I saw a psychiatrist, and I dealt with issues from my childhood around anxiety and some childhood OCD that I'd had. Eventually, they found that I responded to Prozac. And so, I went on Prozac for a period of time. And actually, that addressed the OCD issues as well. So that was quite beneficial, as was the time in the mother-and-baby unit. Without that, I probably would have run myself into the ground just trying to cope with keeping up and running a course that would have had me just collapse in a heap eventually, if not then, in 15 years or so. So, it caused a huge amount of disruption and upheaval. And there could have been things, you know, that could have been done differently, I think, in terms of the care provided, but I'm glad that it all happened because it certainly changed my direction in life and the way that I parent my children now.

Advice to midwives and caregivers

I think having caregivers who listened and could see that I probably wasn't someone that asked for help, could say, 'Hey, you know, I think this is how we can help you.' I think that was important. For people with high-functioning anxiety, this is what I guess I have or had, we don't ask for help because we try to just do it ourselves. And you can't operate like that when the wheels fall off because, in my case, I just had a baby that cried a lot, and I was getting by with so little sleep that I couldn't make those decisions and operate at the level that I normally did. Having carers who listen and respond to needs and who act on concerns that they might have by offering support through a network of services, being aware of what's available for mums that might have a baby who's crying all the time.

When I plot back through that path that I travelled, the support services that were vital were having access to the mother-and-baby unit; having access to a perinatal psychiatrist or a psychologist; having access to multidisciplinary teams who can offer a women's health physio; having a psychology team, psychiatry team, Mothercraft nurses, mother-and-baby nurses or women's health nurses. Also having a GP on board who understands perinatal issues. And then, on top of that, having midwives or caregivers who are receptive and responsive to meeting those needs and being aware of those support services that might need to come into play. Because I'd given birth, and I didn't really know where to turn after that, I think that can be very tricky. I had a home birth, but it can be the same with having a baby in a hospital. You could have wonderful continuity of care through the pregnancy, and then you have your baby, and then you sort of leave the hospital within 12–24 hours if you've had a normal birth. And then you kind of feel as though you're on your own a bit, which can be fine if all goes well. But when there are curveballs, that can be really hard. And it can obviously have a flow-on effect, which is not as good as it was in my case.

Words of advice for students and midwives

My advice would be to learn about mental health. A mental health first aid certificate would be helpful so that you know how to respond appropriately, not even in a time of crisis, but just if you see signs so you know how to respond appropriately. Being aware of services that might be helpful and being sensitive to the needs of someone who presents with anxiety. It can be hard when you've got a mum who does have high-functioning anxiety and just looks like they're totally fine. It's hard sometimes to spot those signs. I guess I'd be looking for someone who's well dressed, has it all sorted, and also has two children in tow that are immaculately dressed. Sometimes looking dishevelled is much more normal than not after you've had a baby.

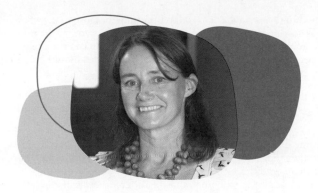

CHAPTER 14

Trish's story

I'm Trish Crampton. I've got twin boys that are 14, identical twins. I'm going to talk a little bit about their birth and my pregnancy and having preeclampsia through that pregnancy.

When I was 5 weeks pregnant I thought that I was probably going to have twins because I was very sick. Then at 7 weeks I found out that I was pregnant and that it was twins, that they were identical. There was one placenta.

The pregnancy was pretty normal except for a lot of morning sickness up to 20 weeks. So not a lot of actual vomiting, but a lot of gagging and all through the day and night and just felt nauseous continuously.

Then at about 20 weeks it sort of stopped. I was pretty healthy. I was working part-time and I felt fine. And then at about probably 27 weeks I started to get a lot more puffy with my ankles and my feet. I was seeing the doctor probably every 2 weeks at that stage, the obstetrician, and he thought everything was fine. My blood pressure was all fine at that stage.

Then I saw him at 29 weeks and I was really puffy, right up to my legs at that stage. And my friend was a midwife and I spoke to her and she said it was still fine. And my blood pressure was okay and he kept checking that and that was okay. And I'd read quite a few books so I sort of knew about preeclampsia and I knew about risks with twin pregnancies.

So from the initial consultation with the doctor he was very adamant that I'd need to have an epidural in place, in case the first twin was born naturally and then there was complications with the second twin, that the needle needed to be in place because it's too hard in between two babies to do that.

So I was really disappointed because I didn't want to go down that track at all. But I could understand it, I thought it was logical. I could see the practical side of it. And I was glad that he had spoken about that, that we spoke about that.

Becoming unwell in pregnancy

So then with the pregnancy, everything was going quite well and I was just getting more swelling. And then in the sort of 29th week it was a hot bout, that week was hot. And I felt very jittery, I felt like I was hungover and a sort of anxious feeling. I didn't really have a headache but I didn't feel well. And I kept in touch with my friend that was the midwife and spoke to her about it. And she said, 'Make sure you put your feet up at night, make sure you're drinking and just rest, take it easy'.

And then I'd been working and I'd been on my feet a lot that day and it was a really hot day again. And that night I just felt it was just, not normal, I just thought this isn't right now. And the swelling had gone up to my waist. So when I laid down I could feel a shift in fluid in my back which didn't hurt but it was very uncomfortable, a revolting sort of feeling. And my thighs and knees and everywhere was swollen at that stage. I rang my midwife and she said, 'I will come over in the morning and see how you go, just have an early night'. So in the morning she came over and took my blood pressure and it was through the roof. So very calmly, didn't tell me that I'd need to probably have the children that day—so I was at 30 weeks at this stage—just said, 'Go to hospital and see what they say'. I was booked in to the public hospital so I went there.

Being admitted to hospital

So we rang the hospital and the midwife that answered the phone sort of questioned whether my source of my reading was correct and accurate. But I insisted that I really did need to go into the hospital and have a proper check and so they accepted that. So I went to the hospital and into the observation rooms of the labour ward and straight away went into sort of panic mode.

I did a urine sample in a cup and it was like orange cordial. So I knew when I did it, I thought that's not good at all. And then, so gave that to her and she just looked and went, oh my god, like, she sort of panicked. My husband was with me at this stage. And then so then she left the room and said I'm going to be giving you a needle. With my reading knew that they'd give me steroids for the lung development.

I said to my husband that that's what they're doing and they think we'll have them today I presume because that's what they do. And he was 'No, no, no'. And then she came back in the room, gave me the injection and said, 'We'll ring your doctor straight away'. And I said, 'Do you think we're going to have them?' And she said, 'Yeah, it's fairly likely'. And then he came and spoke through it all, what was happening and said, 'You've had a tablet and that should bring your blood pressure down, it hasn't dropped yet'. And then eventually it did so that was okay.

So then I went to the observation rooms of the labour ward and they monitored me every hour. So took my blood pressure every hour on the hour. So that was in the morning, I stayed there all day and just managed it. And my blood pressure didn't keep rising so that was good.

That afternoon, the paediatrician from the intensive care came and spoke to me and gave me all the risks. You know, 28 weeks was sort of, to get over the 28-week hurdle was really good. I was 30 weeks so that was a good thing. I'd had the steroids so that was another good thing in favour. And then we did a tour of the NIC. So we went with him and had a look at a 28-week-old baby, a 29-week, a 30-week, looked at all the machines and the different levels of care and he went through all the problems that can occur. So we felt very, we knew what we were up for, we knew what we'd expect, what the babies would look like when they were born, what machines were needed and knew the rooms and all that so that was really good.

Having the babies prematurely

So I lasted 3 days and then one night I had my blood pressure taken and it was high. And so they gave me the tablet. She came back and my blood pressure didn't go down so I had a second tablet. That had happened before. And then the second tablet, a different tablet dropped my blood pressure and this time it didn't drop. So she kept coming back and monitoring and taking it.

So when I came to the realisation that it was all about to happen I was in a scared and, sort of, was hoping that they'd be older than the 30 weeks and 3 days, but it was okay. I cried, and the nurse, the midwife held me and could understand that I was disappointed and scared. And she was very calming with me and was lovely just holding me and making it all seem normal, like she was a good friend even though I'd only just met her.

She called my husband and he came in. So he came into the observation room before we went to the theatre. So he came with me down the corridor to the room. We got to the room, it was pretty scary. There was probably about 12 people in the room. And it wasn't panic, they all seemed very in control of what they were doing, like everyone on their task but it was very busy and everyone moving and it was chaotic. It felt like you were watching a movie rather than being part of it. It didn't feel like reality.

So that's when I saw my doctor in the room and the paediatrician was there that I'd already met in the NIC, so it was good I'd met them before. There was the three anaesthetists that came, that was three women and again they were really nurturing. I was crying and they held me.

Trying to make me feel stronger with it. It wasn't clinical at all. I remember that quite strongly. And then even though the rest was very quick, I think it all happened very quickly it seemed. But I felt like I was in a movie and watching was happening rather than partaking.

So took the first baby very quickly and easily. And the doctor brought him, so I was laying down, brought Oliver to me and showed me, which was nice before he was put into the crib. 'We're taking him to the NIC right now and then we'll get the second baby'. So they did inform me at that stage. And then he went.

So then the second baby was up much higher and it took a long time to physically force to get him out. So they had to really push from this end as well as pull. And I remember my legs going everywhere, not that I could feel them, but I felt like it was very physical getting the second baby out. And it seemed like a long time to get him out, but there was a minute between the two births is what they recorded. But it felt like it was 20 minutes, not sure how long it was. So then they brought Jack and then took him off. And then I don't really remember the next bit.

And then I went to the labour ward and I was in the labour ward for that night in one of their rooms and on quite a bit of medication. I don't remember a lot of it. So my blood pressure didn't drop. You should have the babies and your blood pressure should drop, I'd read that. Well, you should have the epidural and your blood pressure should drop, it didn't. Then you should have the babies and then it should drop further. My blood pressure still hadn't dropped so they were quite concerned about that and I was aware of that happening. I don't know if I had more medication or how they monitored that but they were still taking my blood pressure all through the night every hour.

They kept checking my blood pressure and I knew that they weren't comfortable with what was happening. And a lot of muttering at the end of the bed. And women, the midwives coming in, and you could see them having conversations in hushed tones, you know, 'What are we meant to be doing?' One of the midwives said to me, 'If we had an intensive care unit for mothers here, that's where you would be. But we don't have it so we just have to keep monitoring you hourly and making sure it's all okay.'

Having babies in the neonatal intensive care

So I stayed for the night and the day in the labour ward in the labour room. And then I was in a wheelchair and then I could go into the NIC and see the boys then. So Jack stayed in the most intensive care section for probably 3 days, one-on-one nursing, and then Oliver was in the other one so I held both of them. I held Jack in the most intensive care part briefly. So the nurses that were in the intensive care unit, incredibly special people.

The nurses are very warm in there; they're very empathetic to how you're feeling. They really understand how you're feeling so they'd tell you it was all normal and explain everything and make themselves very available to you if you had questions. And again, a lot of touch, they were very cuddly with us. And for you to, holding them they'd hold you as well and make you feel safe and secure, and very reassuring with what you're doing, what you're doing is right. You know, 'That's great, could put a little bit more here?' or do something, but they'd make you feel very confident with what you were doing which is lovely.

I did a lot of the skin-to-skin contact, so the kangaroo holds. So I'd open my shirt and then we'd take off the little pinafore off the baby and hold him to me. Sort of lying back in a chair so that you have the skin-to-skin contact, they think really helps with the growth of the baby and the heartbeat and the general wellbeing of the child.

So with the skin-to-skin time with the babies, that really helped with the bonding and feeling more confident in holding them and being able to normalise things a little bit. Rather than putting your hands through the crib and touching them that way, it was much nicer to be able to hold them. If you didn't have the oxygen close enough or whatever, you'd get the beeps and whistles and you'd panic and think, 'Oh no, something's happened' but you just bring it closer and they get the whiff of oxygen, they'd pick up again.

I started to express milk at say about day 3. I can't quite remember but early on. So they had an expressing room at the, just near the NIC. And it was a double express machine so you'd feel like a bit of a cow and you'd have the machine going, it wasn't a hand express. And I was able to produce lots of milk which was good. So at first, they'd add fortifying with stuff to the milk which would be to fatten them up. So they used all my expressed milk, I think they had some medication as well but not lots. They didn't have any infections or anything so they didn't need antibiotics which was great. So I just, I expressed when I was at the hospital. I'd just go to the room and express sort of four times a day at the beginning. And we put the milk in the fridge or the freezer. The machines weren't great but it was fine.

Initiating and establishing breastfeeding

So I stayed in hospital for a week, and when the boys were 32 weeks, I'd been home for a little while, they said we'll start to try and start the breastfeeding. They wouldn't have their suckle reflex down pat at all, they were too young still, but might as well start. So I did that at 32 weeks, just once a day. They'd get totally exhausted with anything they did. So any handling, they'd be really exhausted so we'd do that skin-to-skin again.

Then at about 34 weeks, they started to suckle more and take the milk. But again they'd suckle for a little bit and then they'd be exhausted so they were tube fed with my milk the whole time. And then when, to leave the intensive care unit, you need to be fully fed either from a bottle or from breastfeeds, so you had to be off the tube, that's the criteria. So I'd come in sort of three times a day and breastfeed them. And then their other feeds they were fed every 3 hours on the dot. And so they'd have a bottle feed from a nurse and then if I was at the hospital, of the breastfeed.

So they stayed in hospital for 7 weeks. They didn't have any infections or setbacks at all which was a real plus. So they'd just sort of, just got fatter and bigger. They were 1.7 kg when they left hospital. So they'd put on quite a bit for that time. And still tiny but just a bit fatter. So when they left hospital they were fully breastfed.

Taking the babies home

If you have a baby before 30 weeks, you're allowed to have a nurse come to your home and look after you, have the care after that. And I was 30 weeks and 3 days so I was meant to miss out. But because I was having twins and I was very keen to breastfeed, they allowed a nurse to do that, to do the home visits. So she came every day for, I think, a week and then she came twice a week for a couple of weeks after that just to monitor and make sure everything was going okay.

So I did the twin feed with the big feeding pillow, so a baby each side. And I'd always feed together. They were like clockwork, they were every 3 hours fed. And so they'd cry and at 10 minutes before the 3-hour feed, they'd know it was feed-time all through the night and all through the day. So it was very easy knowing. They didn't cry other than the feeds, they were very easy with that. A lot of premmie babies are jittery; they weren't jittery. They were very good sleepers, that definitely helped.

My mum was incredible. I didn't drive, mum wouldn't let me drive for the 6 weeks. So going to the hospital sort of three times a day, mum would drive me twice and then my husband would drive me the once. And she did a lot of the cooking and all of the clothes—washing and ironing, and putting it out and bringing it in—and doing all the sort of jobs for me which was lovely. So it was good that she felt practical that she could help and do something.

Yeah, so it was a nice time for us together. And the nurse that came here, we'd have cups of tea and cake and help with the breastfeeding, but it was a lovely time for all of us. She said she loved her visits here with Mum and myself. And the babies just grew so quickly and, well, that it was exciting to weigh them every time she came. And it was all good, everything just went from strength to strength.

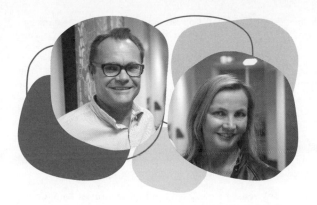

CHAPTER 15

Ali and David's story

Ali: My name's Ali Homer and this is my husband, David. And we'd like to share with you the story of our little girl, Harper.

Our story starts like all parents. We were very excited to discover we were having a baby in late December 2005. It was our first child.

David: There was nothing unusual, every check-up was perfect. Ali's midwife said to her, most times, 'Oh you're so normal, everything's so normal'.

Ali: I was around 32 weeks pregnant. And then I had just noticed over the course of that weekend that there wasn't a lot of lively kicking or very little kicking. But I could feel some movement, so I wasn't particularly alarmed. The next morning I still hadn't felt any kicking and at that point I rang my midwife. And she initially said, 'Look, I'm quite sure everything's okay, but you have called me. And the way that we operate is you've called me so we'd like you to come in and have a check-up.' And we then made our way to the birth centre where I'd planned to give birth.

David: So I picked Ali up from work, fully expecting everything to be perfect. But Ali was, at this stage, quite distressed. And I don't think it was because we knew anything was wrong. It was, I think, simply the first suggestion that something wasn't quite right, that sort of got her very upset. And I remember driving down on that highway, sort of, trying to comfort Ali and saying to her, 'Everything's fine, in 15 minutes we'll be driving back the other way on the highway laughing about how we're crazy, paranoid, first-time parents.'

Ali: When we arrived there, they initially just put a portable Doppler on me. And they did sense a heartbeat but they wanted to use a bigger machine. And then we went into a small room where they used a bigger monitor. And they attempted to find the heartbeat once and then, I'm a bit vague, my memory's quite vague about this part because here's where it all gets dark and quite blurry. But essentially we seemed to have a succession of different doctors coming in trying to complete the ultrasound.

David: And then someone else came in to have another look and the longer—I wasn't looking at the monitor, I was sort of doing my best to comfort Ali—but the longer that there's silence, the worse the news is going to be. And I think there was the two doctors and two midwives, I think, in the room with us. And no one said anything for what seemed like an eternity. And that's actually a really frightening moment.

And I had a glimpse at the monitor and there wasn't any movement. And it was then that they said, 'I'm sorry, it appears your baby doesn't have a heartbeat'. And we were then taken to another, I think it was a dedicated ultrasound suite, for, sort of, confirmation. And again, that silence that goes on forever.

Ali: Yeah, it was a very dark, very dark place then, wasn't it?

David: Yeah, so it was after that, that first sort of confirmation that our baby didn't have a heartbeat, that we were then taken downstairs to another dedicated ultrasound suite. Our midwife that we'd been working with stayed upstairs for, I'm sure she had things to …

Ali: Other women to care for, yeah.

David: So we were in this rather cold, very medicalised ultrasound suite downstairs with someone, with a technician that was lovely but we'd never met and we had no rapport with. Again, there was that long, cold silence, which sort of confirmed to us the worst news. So at this point, Ali was obviously too distressed to walk so she was in a wheelchair. We were both a bit in a daze at that point.

We went back to the room that we were first in. And our midwife sort of just left us both in that room together on the bed. Turned the lights out and called my sister who was in the city. And in what seemed like 3 or 4, 5 minutes, my sister appeared. But it must have been closer to 45 because it's a long drive from the city down to that hospital. Yeah, and then we had to start making some decisions on what we would do.

Ali: What to do next, yeah. At that point I just couldn't fathom what possible options we would have, given that we learnt that our baby had died. I think when you're pregnant you do worry about having a healthy child, and you worry about the obvious things that might go wrong, hoping that they don't. But I can honestly say, and I consider ourselves well educated and well informed, but not one moment out of all those things do you think about the fact that your baby might die.

So when you are given that terrible, terrible news, the thought of what happens next was incredibly foreign to me. And we were very, and I say fortunate now because it really changed our whole experience, we were very fortunate to be given the advice that we should—and we weren't told, it was clearly just a suggestion and advice—that we might want to consider going home, coming back the next day and being induced and go ahead with the birth naturally as I had planned and hoped for.

David: Which, in hindsight, that was the best thing that happened to us. But at the time, I guess it's probably more of a masculine, more of a male way of looking at things, but my thought process was, 'You gotta be kidding me. There's a problem and we're in a hospital. This is exactly where we need to be because you're going to fix this'.

And the thought that we were going to go home just didn't make any sense to me. So I took quite a bit of convincing, because even at that stage I was, 'No, this is wrong, there's a mistake we can confirm, let's stay here and get this fixed'. In hindsight though, it was the best thing that we could do. My sister drove us home to her place, which was a godsend because we couldn't have driven ourselves.

Ali: And I think at that point, whilst I accepted that advice, I didn't for a second really think the thought of giving birth to a dead child, I didn't for a moment think, 'Oh, that's right, I can do that'. It still felt very foreign and very surreal. But I think the way that advice was given to us was very gentle and it was very well thought out, and it obviously gave me the confidence to think I would be able to do it, even though at that point of time I was thinking, like, 'Everything about this is wrong'.

When we got home we made those difficult phone calls to our parents and family and close friends. And it was a really long, that was probably one of the toughest parts of it all that night. It just felt so …

David: Undoubtedly one of the worst nights. There was a lot of long, dark nights to follow that. But that one especially, I mean we'd had all the baby things in the room and just coming to terms that this was actually happening. And quite terrifying for me, and I have no idea how terrifying it must have been for Ali, because I was terrified for the morning knowing that we were going to go back to the hospital. And she would have to go through this ordeal.

Ali: And when we first arrived, we met a doctor who I believe was the registrar, I think. We'd not met him before. And he sort of checked us in and just talked through what we could expect. And we've never seen him again since but his name was Chris and I'll never forget him because he was the very first person amongst, explaining what we could possibly expect, in terms of the induction and the birth.

Before that, his first words to us were, 'I'm really sorry for your loss'. And although we'd spoken obviously to our family and close friends, the fact that a stranger said that, it immediately made me realise that despite this terrible outcome, we were actually still going to have a baby. And even though there'd be no breath, she still would be our child.

David: Stillbirth is still a very difficult thing to talk about. A lot of people really struggle with how to approach it. And that simple phrase 'I'm sorry for your loss' validates all of that stuff that us as parents to an absent child still feel, but is very much, I guess there's quite an archaic view, a tiny minority of people, that if your child didn't draw breath, it's not real.

Ali: It's not really a child.

And I think at that point, considering that we were about to embark on this experience that I had no idea how I would manage, the fact that a stranger said it to me, I can honestly say now, I think it did give me a little bit of strength or it gave me a clear kind of focus. It cleared things up a little bit. So we were in the hospital probably for about 48 hours from beginning to end, wasn't it? I had to be induced. So that all took a little bit of time.

But one of the things that I was at that point still thinking about was, when I thought about actually going through with the birth, I did still feel very scared and very afraid and very unsure of what I would be able to do. But even though that seemed all really difficult, I was still pleased that that's the decision that we had made.

Initially, someone, not our midwife, I can't actually remember who, someone did suggest that we could consider a caesarean. Or we could, as well as the natural birth. And for me, I didn't, the caesarean wasn't something that I ever considered, 'cause I would have thought, I've now just discovered that I'm not going to have the child, I'm not going to be able to take this baby home. And then for it to turn into a medical procedure and then go home with nothing, just seemed awful.

But having said that, the thought of going through with the birth seemed equally as difficult. So I was actually waiting for the third option. That would have been my preference, which, of course, there wasn't one.

So we had time to talk about things that actually were really helpful, although they weren't what we planned. One of them was, we talked about, we started to talk about the funeral that we knew we'd have to have. And that's certainly not something that you think you should be discussing when you're waiting for the birth of your child.

We had other names chosen, whether for a boy or a girl. But we decided at that point, that clearly, it was going to be a special baby so we needed to come up with a new name, which was actually a bit difficult, considering we'd spent a long time coming up with two names and then all of a sudden a third name on the spot.

David: All of a sudden you've got 24 or 48 hours to come up with a new name. But we did. And one of the things that we did in that time when we were in that room together, was we read, I read to Ali from our favourite book, which is *To Kill A Mockingbird*. And the author of that, of course, is Harper Lee. So we decided after a while, that Harper could be a name for a little girl. It would be perfect.

The good thing about that period was we were looked after incredibly well. The midwives were wonderful. Any time we needed anything, they'd come in with hot packs or cold packs or food or everything. They sort of made us feel like …

Ali: They made us feel like they had no one else to look after, which is crazy in a big, busy hospital. But that's how we felt.

David: And I guess the thing about a stillbirth, it's very silent from start to finish. There's no sort of indignant wails of the baby after it's born. And even with the staff, everyone's slightly subdued. So everything that people say to you, you remember. We remember everything people said to us, the wonderful things and the not so wonderful things.

Ali: And I think that's a lot to do with beyond it being silent. You immediately know that you're going to take very limited memory of physical things away from that experience. So you're kind of almost grabbing at things that become part of the story. But we were lucky that we had very few of those comments, that was probably about maybe one or two.

David: The big thing that all the midwives said was those words again that, 'I'm sorry for your loss'. And to someone who hasn't experienced this type of loss, it might sound that they're quite trite, insignificant thing, words. But the reality is again, they just validate what is happening and validate the loss of this life that will never get a chance to.

Ali: They treated us like any other parent that was giving birth. So they didn't take any of the experiences away that, because our child wasn't about …

David: No, we still felt like we were two parents having their first child.

Ali: And at one point, they obviously decided that it would be okay. I can go have my baby in the birth centre, which I'm really grateful for, but I think they were just very careful not to say that's where you're going to be. And I think it was just a much warmer, nicer room, like, it was just nice to get, I mean the other room we had was lovely too, but there was something about that room that I just felt a bit warmer.

David: Well, the other room was a hospital room. Yeah, the first room was in the labour ward, obviously. It's a hospital room.

Ali: It was cold.

David: It's got a hospital bed in it. The bathroom was really cold. It just feels very medical and very clinical, which of course it is. Whereas the birth centre, one of the reasons that we decided before any of this happened to have the baby in the birth centre because it's more of a warmer environment. There's a couch there, the bed's just a regular bed.

Ali: It just felt softer.

David: It didn't feel like we were going through this medical trauma.

Ali: But I remember having our midwife there and I've not obviously been pregnant before, but I could just tell that everything that she did was what she'd do for any other expecting parent. And I can honestly say there was one point during the labour towards the end where I almost, almost, almost forgot that Harper wouldn't have a heartbeat, because I felt I was so engaged in giving birth.

And I think having the strength to do that certainly surprised myself. But at that point it wasn't really about thinking about that. It was just well this is just, this is what we have to do. And then when Harper was born, again we had all the same things that any other parent would do. And Dave, you might want to talk the next bit.

David: I mean when Harper was born, Jacqueline asked if I wanted to cut the cord. And I thought we'd discussed everything in the last 48 hours. But that had never been discussed. And initially I was, sort of, really shocked at that question and then I realised that this is what new fathers do. Which I'm very grateful to her for giving me that option because it would have been very easy in the circumstances to bypass that tradition and do it herself.

But it's one of the few, one of the very few things that I'll ever get to do as a parent for my daughter, so eternally grateful for that. And again it just validated the fact that we'd just had a child. It's just the horrible, the worst outcome possible, but we were still parents of this little girl. And again, it's just that, I keep saying the word validation, but it's just because that was so important and still is really important.

They bundled little Harper up and put her on the bed with us and just left the room for 15, 20 minutes. And that was really important.

Ali: Yeah. I think looking back I do feel very fortunate that our birth experience, the experience itself was so warm and loving and we have very, very fond memories of it. There was the moment where we got the worst news in our lives, and then the birth of our child. They were very distinctly, different events. And I'm very glad they are. Because it means we can actually look back at the birth with some fondness. I'm not sure if that's the right word, but it doesn't feel like this big, black, scary day like the day before was.

CHAPTER 15

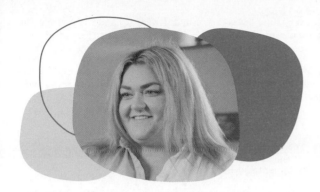

Ashleigh's story

My name is Ashleigh. I'm 29 years old. I have two living daughters, Aria who is 8, Florence who is 4. And I have twin stillborn daughters, Aubrey and Evelyn, who would have been 7 this year.

Twins

When I found out that I was pregnant with twins after the birth of my first daughter, it was quite scary. I was shocked to find out that I was pregnant at all. My daughter was only about 8–9 months old. I was exclusively breastfeeding at the time, so … you know, everyone tells you that you can't fall pregnant when breastfeeding. That's a lie.

I found out that they were twins on Christmas Eve, and it was a massive shock. I cried a little bit but was also very excited. It was a dream of mine to have twins. You know, I always thought that that would be a really great experience. I didn't realise how scary it would be, actually being in that position, but I was excited, nervous, scared.

Losing the babies

In the lead-up to the loss of Aubrey and Evelyn, everything had been actually a pretty good pregnancy. There was lots of monitoring. I was going for ultrasounds every week. I had an ultrasound on a Friday morning, and everything was perfect. The twins were measuring the same. Same size, very close together so there was no concerns at all.

Over that weekend I started to … I guess, feel like I wasn't feeling them move as much. But I wasn't too concerned. I had an anterior placenta with them, so movements weren't as strong as they were in my first pregnancy. And they came much later so I didn't think too much of it.

Come the Monday, I started to get really concerned and that's when I went up to the hospital and … just to get a check-up. And we were given the news that unfortunately both their hearts had stopped.

I think … when we found out that they had passed away, I knew. I already knew. I'd stopped on the way to the hospital and had a big cry in the car. I pulled over, gave myself time to cry about it and then pulled myself together and went up. I just remember them with the Doppler. Trying to find the heartbeat, that they couldn't, so they got out the ultrasound machine. And yeah, there was definitely nothing there. And it was devastating.

I just cried. And my husband cried with me. We didn't know what to do. We just, you know, started to make phone calls. And yeah, there wasn't much more we could do in the moment, I guess.

Having another baby

So, in 2017, I fell pregnant with my youngest daughter, Florence. It was a very, very scary time. I had told my obstetrician, I had told my husband, I had told my friends that I was never having another baby again. I was scared that there was something wrong with me, that I couldn't carry a pregnancy successfully anymore. So, I was terrified.

I wanted more children. I've always wanted a big family. But I was terrified of going through it again, that we would lose another baby.

There was definitely moments of excitement and happiness, that, you know, we might finally have another baby, a sibling for Aria.

But I think the worry definitely over-rid that experience. It wasn't like Aria's pregnancy, which was just very carefree. It was just very stressful at all points. You know, if I didn't feel her move for an hour or so I'd be up at the hospital getting a check-up. And I was very lucky that the hospital was great with me.

During my pregnancy with Florence, I felt very well supported. I used the same obstetrician that I used for Aria and for the twin pregnancy with Aubrey and Evelyn.

She was very caring. She listened to every little concern that I had. She saw me weekly to make sure that I was happy and comfortable knowing that she was still growing, there was still a heartbeat.

I visited the midwives at the hospital quite regularly as well. Every time I was concerned, I went up and they were great with me. They listened to me, they monitored me. I spent a lot of time crying, feeling like I wasted their time. But they were great and gave me a hug and told me that they'd rather me be there every single day, than sit at home worrying.

My husband was by my side anytime I needed him. I have a very close-knit family that, you know, was there to listen every time I was worried about something. Also, all my friends were well aware of what I'd been through and they made sure to check in on me and … yeah, it was great to have that support.

I did do therapy throughout my whole pregnancy. And I do think that that helped me get through it.

The first time that I held Florence when she was born, it was an amazing feeling. I cried, I cried a lot. I cried the whole time I was delivering her. It was just very good to feel that, like again … like just, the feeling of her being put on my chest. Hearing that newborn cry. It's not something that I ever thought I'd hear again.

I had resigned myself to the fact that I'd only have one child. That I would never, you know, feel that again. And it was an amazing feeling.

If I could give any advice for a woman who's lost a baby and wanting another; I would highly recommend therapy. I don't think that Florence would be here today if I didn't go to therapy. It helped me deal with the fact that, you know, it wasn't my fault. Because I think I felt a lot of guilt.

I think opening up and talking about it, when you're ready, is a very important step. I know that it takes time to feel ready to talk again. Still seven years on, and I cry about it when I talk about it sometimes, but it does get better. Talking will make it better.

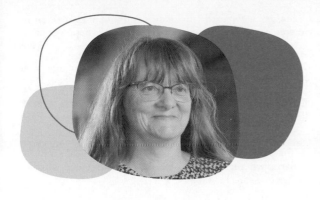

CHAPTER 15

Nikki's story

My name is Nikki Collins and I'm the midwife who coordinates the Early Pregnancy Clinic at the Royal Hospital for Women. And I've been doing that role for approximately 15 years.

Nikki's role in EPAS

My role in EPAS, probably the most important part of my role, is actually support of the women who come through.

Obviously, it's a distressing and difficult time for the women. So, we need to provide them with a comfortable environment, a safe environment, quiet places to be, tissues, answer questions, provide them with information. We provide them with a lot of written information, so that they can always take that away if they need it.

Our role also involves just coordinating the clinic. Organising blood tests, scans, following up on those results and handing over to the doctors who actually see the women who come through the clinic. I also do stats at the end of each day and that looks into the number of women who've been through the clinic, the sort of care that they've decided to take and the outcomes, so that we can actually provide feedback to management and other people who need it; as to how the service is and if we need to do any changes within the service itself.

I chose this particular role a little bit by accident originally. But also finding that this particular part of care for women wasn't very well looked after. When I first started in the UK with EPAS it was a new and emerging service.

The EPAS provides a one-stop shop for women. So, they can come, they have blood tests, they have scans, they see doctors. So, the care is all in one place.

Early Pregnancy Day Assessment Unit

Not everyone woman needs to go to ED. And they can't always provide the support. And they can't always provide all the testing that they need. So EPAS actually provides that for them in the non-acute stage. So those that we can actually have time to sort of scan that don't need anything done urgently; they can come through and be supported. But also, that they've got support after the event. We always give them handouts. I give them my number, my name, so if they feel that they have any questions or any concerns or worries that they can always contact us and that we can follow up for them.

The EPAS at the Royal has set criteria and all hospitals will probably have criteria according to what their facilities are. So, for the women that come through at the Royal, we have women up to 20 weeks of pregnancy who have bleeding and/or pain. We have women who have got confirmed nonprogressive pregnancies. They've been through their GPs and had scans in the community.

We have women who have had miscarriages that have products left behind that need care. And we also have women that come through with early stable ectopics and need further investigation and probable treatment.

Ectopic pregnancies are those where you have a pregnancy outside of the uterus. So, the majority of the time they're actually in the fallopian tubes. And obviously if these rupture then it is a life-threatening situation for women.

But they can be in other areas like the cervix, in the ovary, they can actually be sitting on the bowel. You can even get them in a caesarean scar as well.

They need careful investigation. And then obviously different managements depending on how they present, how big the ectopic is and obviously whatever the woman herself would prefer to have done as well.

But we can also send them for an ultrasound. So that would be vaginal and abdominal scanning, which is really important because with the vaginal scanning you can see things early. So, you can see whether there is a pregnancy in the uterus. And some ectopics will resolve without any further intervention.

So, it's a safe place for them to be monitored and we have everything there. We have the bloods, we have the ultrasounds, we have the doctors available as well.

So, women with pain or bleeding in the first trimester, particularly, very common. Somewhere between 40 to 45% of women will experience those sort of symptoms. But it doesn't necessarily mean that that pregnancy is in trouble.

So, we again do blood tests if we need to. We can do ultrasounds, assess what the pregnancy is doing at that point in time. If it's a very early pregnancy, often we'd need to repeat either blood tests or scan to actually see whether there is an ongoing pregnancy.

And we often do see pregnancies that are fine, and we don't see the women again. But a high majority of the ones that we do see unfortunately will end in miscarriage. But that's what the service is there to provide.

We can also see women that have had miscarriages that have had retained products; a bit of tissue has been left behind. And then we can actually treat them either surgically or medically, or just keep an eye on them and they can let it go conservatively.

We'd also see women who have had terminations of pregnancy, for whatever reason. Because again, they need access to services to follow up with that retained product. And it doesn't matter whether it's been a natural miscarriage or whether it's been a termination, it's a safe place for them to come where we can care for them.

A day in the life of an EPAS midwife

My day in EPAS, we would start with sorting the rooms out, making sure the notes are ready for the receptionists. I also put the radio on, and I also decide which oil I'm going to put in my aromatherapy. I like that because it just makes the environment a little less hospitalised; a little nicer for the women to come through. But it's also a nice environment for me to work into as well.

So I will then triage the women that come through. Have a look at any tests that they've had done so far. Organise blood tests or scans if they need.

If they're women that already have confirmed nonprogressive pregnancies, then I'll actually have a little discussion with them around their options that are available. Answer any of their questions.

So, women sometimes don't need to see the doctor at every visit … when they come through with, for blood tests only, and these are women that we may never have seen where the pregnancy was, but we do need to monitor it to make sure we're not missing a little ectopic.

So, for those, they would see me, I'd organise a blood test, they go home, and then I would ring them later in the day with the results and then organise a follow-up if need be or discharge from clinic depending on what was happening for them.

Women that have recurrent pregnancy loss … difficult, very difficult. Because each pregnancy, they're always going to be worried that this one is not going to be OK as well.

But I think one positive for EPAS is that I will probably have seen these women before. They've been through the system before and I'm hoping that it's a little safer place for them to come. I have seen them, we may have a little bit of rapport going.

So, for these women, we can refer them to recurrent miscarriage clinic which actually is within the department where EPAS is. So, the GPs would need to refer the women and then they can have further investigations and follow-up into possible causes of miscarriage.

All women are offered our counsellor services, at each miscarriage … not just with recurrent loss, but for each miscarriage. And I can make a referral or appointment to the counsellor if they need it.

Top tips for self-care when working with women who experience pregnancy loss

Self-care is really important in this area of care because you are looking after women who have a lot of loss. It's important that you look after yourself.

So, for me, I've been very fortunate that the women that I work with within the department, my work family as I will call them, are there if I need them. And it's so important to realise when you need to ask for help or support.

It may just be them running off and getting coffee for you. It may just be 'I need to close my door for five minutes', but I should be able to have that time and space … it's really important. Organising leave so that you have periods that you're away, that's also very important.

One thing that I do every day is take my dog for a walk, so that's kind of like my meditation, is just to be out on a walk with my dog outside. I'm just away from EPAS and I can forget all of that.

The other thing I tend to do is, I organise myself a massage every month. That's my special treat to help me get rid of stress. Like a lot of neck and back problems, and I think some of that is probably down to a bit of stress. So, it's good just to actually look forward to that every month. I can actually really just treat myself, which is so important.

CHAPTER 16

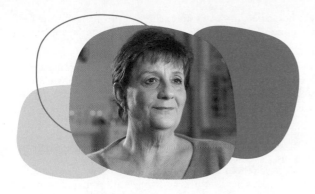

Sandra's story

I am Sandra Emerson and I work in the area of assisted reproductive technology.

Reasons for, and types of, ART

So the most common issues that people face before they come to a clinic is that they may have been trying to achieve a pregnancy on their own, prior to attending a clinic. And the advice is, if you're over the age of 35, you should only try for 6 months before going to see a medical officer about trying to find out the reasons why. And if you're less than 35, it can be a year.

So the most common issue really is age, 'cause women concentrate on their career and then decide to achieve a pregnancy. And it's more difficult to achieve a pregnancy once you're over the age of 37. Your fertility declines each year after that. And often, people aren't going to seek treatment until they're 40, 42, 44. And often the pregnancy is far more difficult to achieve at that time.

Often there's reasons of male problems with sperm production. Often there might be male medical issues that might be an issue about achieving a pregnancy for them. And also, most commonly, if you're overweight, it's more difficult. So they say that if you're over 100 kg in weight, then it's more difficult to achieve a pregnancy. So it might be as simple as just getting advice on losing weight. But there's a great gamut of reasons why people might not be able to achieve a pregnancy. But most commonly it's age.

So the most common types of ART, I think most people think ART is just IVF. But assisted reproductive technology can run from just monitoring a cycle for a couple, who are trying to achieve a pregnancy, and maybe they have irregular cycles. So it's difficult for them to time when they're ovulating. And a lot of clinics will do cycle monitoring. There's a natural cycle with using the husband's sperm that has been prepared for intrauterine insemination, timed at the right time of the cycle.

There's clomiphene citrate, which is an oral medication which they take at the beginning of their period. And that encourages the growth of follicles by stimulating the pituitary gland to increase more FSH and LH. And then having intrauterine insemination, often can have follicle-stimulating hormone injections and insemination. And they're probably the most simple types of ART, if you can call it simple having to inject yourself every day.

Then you move into the IVF area. And so that is often very time consuming, and some types of cycles can take up to 6 weeks. And it starts with decreasing the woman's hormones to put them into the menopause really. And then starting to build their hormones up and increasing the follicular development. And then egg harvesting. And then putting back an embryo about 5 days later, after the egg collection.

Other cycles can be included in that is doing pre-implantation genetic diagnosis for many women, if they've done many cycles that have failed. Often they'll test the embryos and they'll just remove one cell and test it for any genetic disorders that may be affecting the cell, 'cause as we get older, women's eggs are not as good as they were when we were 20. So they more commonly will have abnormalities. So lots of women are choosing to have that as well now.

And then, of course, if there's a problem with sperm production, often they have to harvest the sperm from the testicles of the men. And that has to be coordinated with the cycles. And then that testicular tissue is frozen and they harvest the spermatids from there and use those to inject into the egg. So it's quite complex, and depending on what type of treatment you're having, depending on what is your problem with achieving a pregnancy, most commonly there's this terrible grey area called 'unknown'. It just falls into this grey area of 'we don't know why you're not achieving a pregnancy'.

So, often the cycles can be changed from cycle to cycle to try and improve them. But often it can be quite complex and very wearing on women to be injecting themselves, taking nasal spray to put them in the menopause, to be injecting themselves every day, to have a light anaesthetic to do the egg harvesting. And then 6 weeks down the track, finally you might achieve a pregnancy, and you may not. And then you're sort of having to start all over again. So it's quite emotionally draining.

So as far as fertility preservation, that's certainly an area that's increasing. And so many younger women now are going to clinics and exploring the option of freezing their oocytes, and putting them away for the future. Particularly if they're in their early thirties and they don't have a partner, or they're not expecting to try and achieve a pregnancy in the next few years, then certainly now, what they're doing is they're coming in, having a stimulated cycle, they're having an egg collection and those oocytes are then frozen.

And so that, in years to come, if they would like to achieve a pregnancy with a partner or they're going to use donor sperm, then those oocytes are there. They may be 10 years older, but the oocytes are the age that they were when they were collected, which increases your chance of pregnancy. So that's becoming more common. Young women are coming in to freeze their oocytes for future preservation of their fertility. So that's certainly increased in the last 5 years.

What the couple has to go through

So the physical side, I guess, of the treatments are that often some cycles, as I said, can take up to 6 weeks. That's quite a long time. Particularly when you're trying to work, you often haven't told anybody. And you're on medications that cause wonderful side effects like bloating, breast tenderness, nausea, extreme tiredness and you're still trying to work. So often it will start at a cycle. And on day 20, you go in for a blood test on what's called an agonist cycle. They check that you've ovulated and then you start a nasal spray, which drops all your hormones down to baseline. So you get the effects of the menopause, night sweats and not feeling terribly fabulous.

And then they start. You do daily injections of hormones, of follicle stimulating hormone, and they might be quite small doses or they may be quite large doses. The most common side effect from those is really extreme tiredness, the bloating as the ovaries increase with more follicles being developed. And so you get abdominal discomfort and you don't sleep terribly well. And often people find that extremely wearing and quite challenging to fit in their normal routine, as well as trying to do all of that.

And then you have the egg harvest. And there is that possibility that you'll get ovarian hyperstimulation. Everybody gets a mild form of that. So your ovaries are very enlarged from the numerous follicles that are being developed from the medication. So, again, afterwards breast tenderness, abdominal discomfort, bloating, often can increase at that time, so really, you're certainly not feeling terribly well after all of those drugs.

And so it's very difficult to try and maintain a normal life for some women, not all. And so trying to find that support and emotional support from the nursing staff in the clinic, that's very much where they get a lot of support from on a day-to-day basis. And their partner. Sometimes they won't have told anybody they're doing the treatment.

It still tends to be something women don't talk a lot about often with their family. They might with their girlfriends, but often not with their family. So they really have to rely on the husband. And that's very difficult because he's not there every day. Except for the injections, he's not receiving the injections.

But often, what happens is, is that they'll come in with lots of questions. And we must never forget the husbands. He's as much a part of that treatment as the woman. But he's at the other end, at the trying to deal with the side effects of that medication at home. And a lot of the husbands do the injections for their wives. So that sort of makes them feel involved in the process.

The emotional side of having treatment is that you're always, perhaps, not feeling very well on the drugs, but also, you're trying to achieve a pregnancy. You may have been trying for some years on your own. So the more emotional side comes after the egg pick up, I think, and then when you have the embryo transfer. Up until there, you're going to the clinic every day, or every other day, maybe every 2 days or every 3 days. So you've got that contact with the nursing staff in the clinic.

After the embryo's been transferred, you don't go back to the clinic for 2 weeks. So you're sort of a bit abandoned, I think, in many ways. That you don't have that contact every other day with the nurses. Although they do ring you about a week after, to see how you are. And of course, they're always available.

So emotionally, often what women say is, the slightest pain, they run to the bathroom to see if their period is there. Or they get a small spot of blood and they just think the whole thing hasn't worked. And so it's the last 2 weeks, I think, is terribly emotionally draining on women because they're just waiting, waiting and waiting. And if they get their period, that's absolutely devastating because the cycle hasn't worked.

And so, I remember one woman who rang me up and asked me what we'd done to her cycle. 'I haven't got my period, what have you done?' I said, 'Do you think you might be pregnant?' and she said, 'Why would you think that?' Like she just thought we'd ruined her cycle. Didn't think that she could be pregnant. And I thought isn't that a sort of strange way to look at it. She assumed that something had happened to her cycle because she never thought she'd achieve a pregnancy.

And I've had someone, when I was taking their blood to do a pregnancy test, say, 'I don't know why you're bothering to do this. I'm not pregnant'. And in actual fact, she was.

So they actually never get to the point of thinking they actually will get pregnant. It's too hard to go over that line and possibly hope that it's going to work. And yet they have this hope up until that time. So it's sort of this real mix of feelings, I think. They hope and hope and hope. And then when the period doesn't come, they still don't think that they could possibly be pregnant, especially women who've been trying for a long time. And so often, that's a really difficult time for women, I think, especially emotionally. So if they're very emotional, it has that impact on their partner as well.

The cost of ART

For many couples, especially if they've been trying for many years, a cost of a cycle will vary from clinic to clinic, and depends on who you go to. There are a few low-cost clinics now available in Sydney, where they do basic IVF. So it's only for families who have IVF, straight IVF, not intracytoplasmic sperm injection, where they insert the sperm into the egg. It's just pure IVF. So when the egg and the sperm are put together and they do it all itself. And so that's now available. There's quite a number of clinics popped up in Sydney now that have that low-cost model.

If you're requiring anything like intracytoplasmic sperm injection, prenatal genetic diagnosis, all of those things, they of course cost more money. And often what happens is people will continue and continue. And I've known people to add to their mortgage to do more cycles. And often that's very stressful to do that.

And so if you do one cycle or two or three, you do get a Medicare rebate. But certainly, it can be very expensive depending on what you're actually having done. Because pre-implantation genetic diagnosis costs more, embryo transfers then you pay for, and also if you're having other medications which aren't covered, that's an extra financial strain.

So often, it's very difficult to find the money. Some families lend them the money, other people, as I said, take out mortgages, people will save up just to do one cycle. Or they'll do one cycle and then have to stop and save up again. And so depending where you go, will depend on how much the cost is. So each clinic will have a different cost.

If it doesn't work, often people are under that financial pressure. They may not have that money to pay for another cycle. Often, even if they do, they often do cycle after cycle and often won't go on holidays. Because they think, well if I go on holidays and I don't do a cycle, that one might have worked. And so they won't change jobs often because they think, well if I change jobs and I can't then get time to go to the clinic, then I might have missed a cycle that would work.

And so often they certainly will just do cycle after cycle, if they can afford it because they think if that one will work, then I don't want to stop. But it can be very emotionally and financially draining to try and find that money, maybe every 8 weeks. And so it can be quite challenging, I think, for many couples.

I think, even in the area that I work in, and I work in both areas, so I'm in many ways extremely lucky that I get to see women who've gone through IVF. I may have even looked after them. And then they come through and I may meet them again, for whatever reason during their pregnancy. And I guess that came to the fore the other day when I looked after a lady, who had a baby. And she's sitting there with the baby in her arms and she said to me, 'Sandy, I still keep waiting for someone to come and take this baby away and telling me it's not really mine'.

And even after all of this, that still hit me in the face that women still can feel that. If they've been trying for many years, they still don't believe that this is their baby when it's finally there with them. And I guess it just reminded me, above everything else, just remember, that even then, they need that little bit of extra support and encouragement. Because they still think someone's going to come and take that baby away.

The midwifery care

When you're doing a booking visit and you get to the point of asking, have they had assisted reproductive technology, it's more than just ticking a box. Because if someone's had one cycle of, say IVF, or one cycle of stimulated cycle with insemination, their coping mechanisms for a pregnancy and how they approach a pregnancy are very different to someone who's had 10 cycles of IVF.

And often women who've taken a long time to achieve a pregnancy will be much more anxious than someone who's had one cycle. Often they'll say, they don't count their chickens before they're hatched, because they always think something is going to go wrong. 'My body failed me, I had to get this treatment to get pregnant, so now what's going to happen with this pregnancy?'

So they often will only take in small amounts of information. Often when we meet pregnant women for the first time, we hand them a whole bunch of things to read in a packet. Most people never read half of it. But you can't do that with someone who's had lots of IVF because you have to layer your information.

And so I always say, IVF is more than just a tick box or ART is more than just a tick box when you're doing a booking. It's important you stop then and say to the woman, 'Well, how was that for you? How many cycles did you do?' and try and explore what her level of anxiety is about this pregnancy.

Because often these women won't have ever thought that they will achieve a pregnancy, so often getting to that point increases their level of anxiety again, but in a different area. And so they often don't know a lot about pregnancy, what's needed or expected, and tests and things in pregnancy. So that often makes it another challenge for the midwife who might be booking them in to care for them. But they just need to remember, to just stop and ask a few open-ended questions like, 'How was that for you?' Because you will get a lot of information from the woman about that.

Often women will go overseas and have treatment. And they often have difficulties disclosing that information, so that's really important if you're that woman's primary caregiver as the midwife, that you know about that. And that way will allow you to tailor your care appropriately to that woman.

A day in the life of Sandy

So a typical day, I guess, in the day of a nurse that works in a reproductive medicine clinic, is … it's an early start: 7 o'clock if you work during the week, 8 o'clock on the weekends. So typically you have women and their husbands coming through for, perhaps, just blood tests. And often they have lots of questions. Or they might be having a blood test and an ultrasound. And the nurses perform the ultrasounds and take the bloods. They also might have, typically for those women who are having a cycle where they're doing intrauterine insemination, that the nurses also do the intrauterine insemination for the woman.

So it's quite varied, often very challenging dealing with everybody's emotions during the day and questions. And being there to support those families as they come through. And then, of course, you deal with all of the results, speak to the medical staff about those results, change the treatment perhaps, for the following few days, increase their drugs, decrease their drugs. You might need to bring them back the next day or in a few days, so you make up all their following appointments.

And then you're conversing with the women about what their results mean, what that means for the cycle, depending on what sort of cycle they're doing. 'Is that good?', that's often a question. 'Is that a good result?' So, often that's really important that you're conveying exactly how that is for her in her cycle. Often it's difficult though if there are problems with stimulating the woman. You're having to let her know, perhaps, that this cycle isn't going the best and you're going to cancel the cycle. Often that's quite devastating for the women.

And the other thing is if you're planning to do the egg pick-up in 2 days, being very specific about instructions of when to take certain injections. What time they'll be coming in to have their egg pick-up done. And then, when their husband's expected. So it's very, very challenging. It's a great place to work.

CHAPTER 16

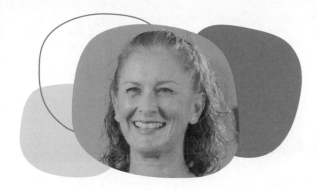

Robyn's story

My name is Robyn. I'm a single mother of twins and I chose to become a single parent through an anonymous donor when I was 39 years old.

I never thought in my whole life that I would be nearly 40 and still single. And there was always just something missing in my life. I'd always desperately wanted to be a mother. And then getting closer to the end of my 30s, I was like, 'I either I make this decision now to go through a donor and have a child on my own, or I go through the rest of my life being a single woman with no children'.

So, I started to talk to some people that I knew who had already gone down this same path, and they gave me the confidence to actually do it as well. And it took a lot of research for me. And it took a lot to get my head around. And I spoke to my family as well letting them know that this is what I really wanted out of my life, and they were very supportive. I think they obviously had their concerns as well about how I was actually going to do this on my own. But being such an independent person all my life anyway, and travelling the world by myself, moving all around ... I didn't see it as anything different to what I had already done. I had always just been so used to doing things on my own and being so independent.

So, I made some appointments to go and see a fertility specialist down in Sydney. At the time ... so this was just over 10 years ago that I started my journey, and a local fertility group here were not as supportive for a single person to go through having a child on their own. They were more accepting of same-sex couples or heterosexual couples that were just having difficulty falling pregnant. But not so much for a single person. So, I went to a fertility clinic in Sydney, and I had a lot of trips down in Sydney to different appointments. Consultations, counselling sessions, and that wasn't to sort of see whether I was mentally stable enough to become a parent on my own. It was more about me understanding the legal side of things that by going through an anonymous donor, the donor has no legal right or anything to the child and I can't ask for any type of monetary support from them as well.

So, with knowing all of that, I was still obviously really keen just to get started on the whole process. I had a consultation with the fertility specialist, and I said that I wanted to fall pregnant as naturally as possible without actually just having a partner to conceive that way. So, we spoke about intrauterine insemination, or IUI, and we chose that path for me. And then if that wasn't going to work then we would look at IVF. So, with the intrauterine insemination process I needed to have a series of scans and x-rays. I needed to have a set of x-rays done where they actually placed dye through my fallopian tubes just to make sure that there was no blockages whatsoever. Because they would not do IUI on somebody if it was not going to be a successful process. So, luckily for me, I was all completely healthy in my reproductive system. So that was great.

So, the first cycle I had they monitored me very, very closely. So, they want to know the date of your last period. They want to track you through blood tests very, very closely. Just to see the levels of, I'm guessing, your hormones. And then they gave me a list of donors they had in the clinic at that time. And I could get onto a website and look at the details from that donor. So, it gave me a lot of information and that was hair colour, eye colour, skin tone, their interests. I just got about a 10-page profile on my donor. And that was really important to me, that I had quite a lot of information for one day when my children start asking the questions 'who is my father' or ... and I don't even refer to the donor as a father. It's a donor. I can give them that profile and they can see all the information. And the donor had actually written a really nice little piece in his profile as well, about why he was doing this. And that was something that really drew me to that particular donor. The donor profile also had information about his siblings, his parents, his maternal grandparents, paternal grandparents and aunts and uncles. So, that has given me quite a cross-section of genetics, really. That I can actually now see some of that coming through my children because I know it's not from me.

So, when it got to the point that I was going to have the treatment, I had to give myself a trigger injection in my abdomen. And that obviously triggers the eggs to release. And then I need to be down at the clinic by a certain time on a certain day for them to do the procedure. So, the procedure itself to me was just like having a pap smear done. And then they just threaded a very fine tube through my cervix and into my uterus, and then inserted the semen that way.

Unfortunately, the first time didn't work for me. But I had that approach that well this obviously isn't the right cycle for me. So, I spoke to the specialist again and they decided that they would give me a stimulant of Clomid. And I needed to give myself an injection again in my abdomen every evening at the same time. Just to get my eggs to a level of maturity.

So, I gave the injections and that was hard. That was hard for me being a single person and not having the support of a partner there to sort of 'come on, you can do this'. And I remember sitting on the side of my bed one night thinking 'right, what's more important, do I not give myself this needle because I just didn't like it or am I still going to go on through my life without the chance of having a child'. So, I just did it. And I didn't think anything of it after that. I just knew that this is what I needed to do to help me achieve this dream. And I went down to Sydney for my treatment, and I fell pregnant.

So, then I had to go for a blood test a couple of weeks after that just to confirm the pregnancy. I had already started to feel soreness in my breasts and things like that anyway. Just little symptoms like that and I was like … 'oh, am I, aren't I? I don't know, this hasn't happened before, I'm not sure'. And I remember I was at work, and I used to always go into the toilets and just be like, 'oh yeah, they're still sore, maybe this is it, maybe this is working'. So, I was just like 'please let this be it'.

So, I went for the blood tests and then they rang me that afternoon and confirmed the pregnancy. And they said that my hCG levels were really high. Which then I was like, hmm, what does that mean? And they said it doesn't necessarily mean there are twins, but the levels are quite high. So, then I had to go for a 7-week scan and that was when I found out that I was having twins. So, that was a bit of a shock to the system. I think in the back of my mind I always knew that that was what was going to happen for me. But then, having that confirmation scan I was like 'oh my gosh'. And my sister was with me as support during that scan. And she went, it's OK, you can do this. You can do this; we can do this. It takes a village. And we will do this. You will be fine. And then after that, I knew that it didn't matter what happened. Everything was going to be all right.

So, that first 12 weeks was quite nerve wracking, I guess. Like it would be for any new parent in any pregnancy, having to go for the nuchal translucency scans. And I remember sitting there saying to my mum, what if something is wrong? She said, well if something's wrong, we'll just deal with it at that time. Because it's really hard, as positive as you can be, it's really hard not to have those little doubts in the back of your mind until you really know that everything is OK and that your babies are healthy. So, I had that scan. Everything was looking great. Then I started to show so I needed to tell people because I wasn't just trying to keep it really low key. But two babies, it was a bit hard.

Because of my age and also having the multiples, I was classed as high-risk. I had just such wonderful care through those ladies. I had regular appointments. They made everything available to me on how my pregnancy was going and then what it might look like when it came time to deliver my babies.

I kept myself really fit during my pregnancy. I was swimming, I was doing yoga, and then I just went, 'I just need to go in and do what I need to do'. And I knew in my mind that I could do it.

I had complete trust in my midwives. They listened to me. If I said, 'no I don't want to go book in at this time, I want to keep going'. We set the goals, it was to get to 32, 34, 36, and we kept getting past these goals. I think it was about 34 weeks and they said, 'OK we're going to book you in for an induction, so if you have not had these babies by this date, you're going to be induced.' I'm like that's fine. So, we got to 34 weeks. Everything was fine. The babies were healthy, I was healthy. And my focus was making sure that they were there for as long as possible. That I could keep them safe, keep them in a safe environment, help them grow as much as possible too. I really wanted to avoid them having to go to NICU if they were going to be healthy.

I ended up being induced at 38 weeks, 5 days. So, having both head down enabled me to have a completely natural delivery of my babies. And that was something that I had spoken to my midwives about as well. They wanted to know what sort of pain relief do you think you might want and I just said, 'I don't know, I really don't know, I just want to see how it goes on the day.' I didn't even know how I was going to manage labour, let alone trying to think about what type of pain relief I was going to have. So, I just made sure I knew what was available to me. And made sure my midwives knew that I just needed to go with the flow on that day.

I had made the decision from early on that I didn't want a birth plan. To me, I feel that birth plans set you up for something and then if it doesn't work out it can really make you feel maybe like you've failed in some way if it hasn't gone to plan. And this is something that can't go to plan. All I knew is that women do this every day. This is what my body is designed for and that's what I'm going to go in there and do.

So, I had a lot of support from my family. And I think even some of my extended family were a little bit shocked by my decision. And I think a lot of it was more around 'why is she doing this, why would she want to do this on her own, how is she going to support these babies?'

And most of the people that know me really well knew that this was something that I always wanted. So, they were very supportive, and they were wonderful. The wider community, in some ways, I felt slightly judged. Not that I let that worry me because I felt that they weren't direct people in my life. The silly comments you would hear people say about it, about going through a donor. And if I could just expand on that a little bit, it was things like, 'oh well don't you want to know how many babies your donor has fathered?' I'm like, no, that's irrelevant to me. I don't care. 'You sure, you don't want to know?' And I was like, 'I don't care'.

But yeah, I think a lot of people, most people were really accepting. And there's always going to be a few that sort of say a lot of strange things and sort of judge you on that. But I just got to that point in my life where I just went, 'I just want to surround myself with those people that do support me, that do understand me' and that's what I did.

So, I did go to one parenting group just focused on multiple births. I think there was maybe ten couples there and I was the only single parent. And I just went on my own and I made some ... two mainly, wonderful friends just from going to that group. And then we all became part of Multiple Birth Group as well. And that group was an absolute saving grace for me. So, after I had my babies, I went to my first group catch-up with them when they were 8 weeks old. And I could've skipped the whole way home. Because I knew I wasn't alone in this. I was talking to other people that were going through exactly the same experiences that I was going through. Which, people can say, 'oh I've had a baby, I know what it's like'. But I had my sister who has got three children, I had my mum who had two of us and I was living with my parents after I had my kids and mum was like 'it's completely different when you've got two babies in one go'.

So, these families that I became friends with through that group were a tremendous support during those really early years, when you've really got no idea what you're doing. And we're still friends to this day, nine years later.

Since I've had my children, I have come across a few other single women who have spoken to me about my journey and their interest in going down the same path as I did. And I'm always open to talking to women about this because I think as a woman, we are so lucky that we have this opportunity to be a parent on our own more so than what men are. And the advice that I give to them is, make sure you have all the information that you think you need to know. Try not to plan your whole birthing, you know, the day that you give birth and have a plan what it's going to be like. Because it's just so different for everybody.

I always recommend that they try and stay as fit and active as they can during their pregnancies. Because I feel that that helps during delivery, and also mentally and emotionally at the end of it. And I also say to them that, just make sure you're doing this for you. Make sure you're doing it for the right reasons and not because it's what somebody expects of you. Or what society expects of you. And the rest of it will come. Just surround yourself with supportive people and you will get through it. There are days where you don't think you will, and you will cry, and you feel so emotionally, mentally and physically drained. But you do get on with it. And you just have to look at your children every day. And there's always challenges but the good always outweighs the bad. And it's such a wonderful, wonderful experience.

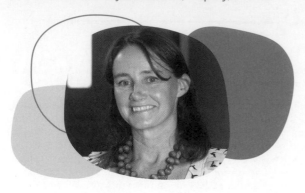

CHAPTER 17

Trish's story

I'm Trish Crampton. I had a vaginal birth after a caesarean section with twin boys that were born at 30 weeks. So I fell pregnant 5 years after the boys were born. They were born at 30 weeks with an emergency caesar. I was really keen to have a vaginal birth with my next baby. I went back to the same doctor that I'd had with the twins and he was very adamant that I should have another caesar. I'd already had one and that was safer for me and safer for the child to go down that track.

I wasn't comfortable with that. I didn't feel that that had to be the way. I did some research and spoke to a friend that was a midwife and she actually had a pamphlet that I took back and spoke to him further about it.

Deciding to try for a vaginal birth after a caesarean

I had a very good scar and that I'd like to try for a vaginal birth and then if emergency came into it then, if it needed to be then that was okay. But I'd like to definitely try. So he agreed to that. But it was a lot of negotiating, a lot of pushing on my behalf. He certainly didn't want to go down that track and made it known.

My friend that is a midwife that I spoke to about it, she had another friend that was studying midwifery. And she needed to do some follow-ups through a pregnancy, so she came with me which was really, a really good experience. So she came with me to the obstetrician appointments and met the doctor and said that she would be at the birth, if she was able to. He was very informative with her. So he would talk through the ultrasound and explain things to her. I think she had a good experience with him.

The doctor was good with explaining things to me as well. I found him with the last pregnancy and birth to be informative. He likes you to know and he's very upfront with everything so he would talk through the pros and cons or he'd say why he was doing things and what he was doing every step of the way always, which was great.

Another thing the doctor did bring up, that he would not let me go over term. He gave a specified time. I think I was allowed to be 5 days overdue and after that it was to be a caesar, not even to be induced. He was very keen for a caesar at that stage so I felt like I had to negotiate with him quite often through the pregnancy and then again through the birth.

There was, it felt like there was some give and take always, 'Okay, so you're allowed to do this, but then at that point, you're not allowed to'. It's probably just a personality thing with him but that was okay.

It was a very normal pregnancy, so got to full-term and then I was a little bit overdue, so I was like 2 days overdue. Had a little, thought I was going into labour, or did go into labour, but it didn't eventuate. And then I was to see him again. I asked for a stretch and sweep. And he would not do that, he said he doesn't do that and was very black and white about it, that that was a 'No', and not to be discussed, and he wouldn't negotiate on that.

From that stage I had a stretch and sweep from my midwife friend because he wouldn't. I didn't discuss that with him. I didn't tell him that's what I was doing. I had that done one evening and then that night I went into labour. I stayed at home as long as I could. My children were in the house, I just wanted to get out of the house.

I suspected I wasn't going to go into having the baby very quickly, but I wanted to get to the hospital so we did. Got to the hospital and I hadn't dilated. And the doctor came and he broke my waters. It was in the morning and he said that he would give me till midday. If I wasn't 10 cm dilated at midday, I was having a caesarean. So again, he was very black and white; that was the terms of the agreement.

Having a vaginal birth after caesarean

So I had till midday to be 10 cm dilated and he wasn't going to come back before. And it was very cut and dry. And it was like it was an agreement but I didn't really have any say in the matter at all. It was, if I wasn't, I was having a caesar, that was his decision and I didn't feel like I had any say in it. You can't really force your body to become 10 cm dilated. It was out of my control, but I got there.

So when I got to the hospital, my friend that was the midwife came with me, just as a support person, not as a professional midwife. Another midwife from the hospital arrived and spoke and my friend set up the, put on a belt to see, monitor the heartbeat and all that. So she knew that we were coping very well on our own and she left us pretty much for the day. I just progressed through the labour quite well and quite quickly from that stage when he broke my waters.

The midwife that was studying to be a midwife came as well. So it was really nice having familiar faces and people that I knew well, my husband knew well, in the room. I knew the doctor wasn't coming back till midday which very much suited me, so I could just try and do the best to get to that stage that for when he came back I could go with a natural birth.

And it was hard work. It was labour but it was very comfortable. I felt very comfortable in my surroundings and with the people around me. My husband was there the whole time as well. And it was sort of like a team effort; we were all working together for this. My husband's quite competitive so it was sort of like, we're racing against the clock and yeah, we're getting there, we can do this together. It was quite a team effort I felt; I wasn't on my own battling on. And definitely having the people that I knew and loved around me was really good. I think that helped the labour progress.

Giving birth

So pretty much 12 o'clock on the dot, the doctor arrived and sort of, put the gloves on and was gowned up and all that. And then examined me and he was really surprised. He said, 'Well, you're 10 cm, you've got what you wanted sort of thing. We're ready to go, we'll try for the vaginal birth. You don't have to have the caesar'. So it all went normally. It was very quick and easy for most of it.

I did feel, it definitely changed, the air changed with just the midwives and two friends to then him arriving. He was in control, he was taking over. It was okay, all systems on now. Towards the end, the baby, little baby girl, he used the ventouse and vacuumed her out which may or may not have been necessary. Probably not, but that was just how it was.

The doctor was good with the student midwife, my friend. He did speak to her and had her involved with the delivery which was good. Then he did an episiotomy as well which was probably not necessary, but again didn't discuss it with me. It was just, this is what's happening. But the doctor was very chuffed when she was born and he was very much, 'Well, that's what you wanted and it's been a really good result'. And he seemed quite pleased with himself as well.

She came straight onto me. She was a big, healthy baby compared to the 30-week-old twins. Screaming lungs and very fat and healthy, so that was all really lovely. My husband burst into tears. But the doctor was quite softened by it; he's got five children himself. And you could see he was quite emotional about it as well, which was nice to see that other side of him. That wasn't the cut and dry, you must have the caesarean. So, yeah, it was a good ending.

So when I did, the baby was on me and it was all over, I couldn't believe there was so much pain and then just no pain. And just so elated and just felt like I was on an absolute high. My husband was crying, we were all crying and it was, yeah, such a great feeling I felt really. So I held her and then straight away I went to breastfeeding.

The midwife that was a student, she gave the vitamin K needle and that was the first baby that she'd ever given the needle to and that was all exciting for her too. It was a lot of firsts for all of us so it was exciting. Yeah, it all went well, so then the breastfeeding from there just went very well. She knew what to do and there was no problems at all with her latching on, everything was very easy with breastfeeding. So that was good.

Everything just felt so right

When I had Annabelle it was just so easy and it just felt so right. I spent a lot of time just holding her. So just holding her and looking at her and really enjoying the moment, and thinking this is how it should be.

I was in hospital for the 2 days I think and then just came home. I felt with the caesarean before, the recovery and the pain, felt that dragging, pulling feeling for a long time. And felt nothing with the, I was very swollen with having Annabelle, but I was very, felt fit and healthy and so many happy drugs sort of in me, natural. I was on a real natural high for a long time.

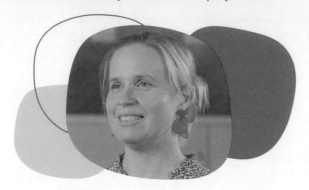

CHAPTER 18

Elise's story

So, my name is Elise and I'm a mother of two beautiful girls. I had my babies 10 years ago and 8 years ago. And I chose to have those babies through a continuity of care model and through that I decided I was going to birth my babies in water.

I decided to have water births mainly as a form of pain relief … was what I decided. I didn't actually plan on birthing necessarily in water to start with. But because I chose to have my babies at home, water was mainly the only option I had. And I had a small house and a corner bath, and a birth pool was an option for pain relief.

First water birth

So, for my first baby it was a longer labour because the baby was posterior. And without even knowing, using water allowed me to manipulate my body into like, a wave … like a snake, so that I could rotate my baby. I really liked birthing in my little safe cocoon, so to speak. Because when I'm in pain I don't like being touched. So, my pool was big enough that they could get to me but also big enough that they weren't in my space. So, I guess that's why I really liked that side of it. I also liked being buoyant and not having that weight of a heavy belly as well.

So, birthing in the birth pool that I had, it had an inflatable bottom. So, it allowed me to squat in a position where I was able to actually touch my baby's head and I was the first person that touched my baby. And then without even planning it, I just reached down and brought my baby up, and that was amazing. It was just me and my baby in that moment. I couldn't even tell you who else was in the room. It was just amazing.

And my husband just remembers me lifting this beautiful baby up and me just going, 'oh my god, it's a pink one'. Like, I couldn't even say it was a boy or a girl or what it was. And it was so calm. Like, she just was on my chest looking at me and I don't even know how long it was until she cried. But it was calm, there was just that moment of pure silence. It was just beautiful.

Second water birth

That's why I chose then to use water for my second baby. As a form of pain relief more than anything. Because I did try to get out of the birth pool, and I really didn't like it. I felt heavy, I felt … I didn't feel at peace or grounded or whatever. Like, the water was my happy place, and it has always been a place I like to go to if I need to feel at peace or relaxed. I'll have a bath or go to the beach and be by the ocean. So, for me the water was something that meant that I could remain calm, I suppose, and not frightened.

I'd also had care through a continuity of care model. And they had talked a lot about water births and the benefits and the research behind it. So that you would have a quicker labour if you used water immersion, which is also the shower. But I didn't have a very big hot water system, so once I filled that bath … pretty much topped it up with boiling water. And it's also for perineal integrity basically. There is good evidence for water birth, protecting your perineum. So, that was why I also decided to have a baby in the water.

I did get quite hot at times because I was working hard. So, just being mindful of staying hydrated I think was important because I had forgotten about that. So, being offered drinks was really helpful. And keeping cool. I also liked it because, for me, I didn't like noise, so I put ear plugs in my ears and I just blew bubbles into the water. So, that was how I got through my labours was just blowing bubbles in the water. Which I guess I couldn't have done if I wasn't in the water. And sometimes if I felt overwhelmed, I took the ear plugs out and I just put my head under the water. And yeah, that helped.

I couldn't have a baby without water though. I will say that. I don't know how I would cope if I didn't have the option of water. That's my go-to.

So, I didn't have any examinations, so I didn't have to get out for that.

I did have to get out for the toilet once. I do remember that, and I did not like it. So, after that, if you were going to put your hands in the water, it was at your own risk.

Some of the things that I really enjoyed about the bath was I had the benefit of being buoyant. But also allowing access to my back for massage and pain relief that way. Because I was able to lean forward, feel supported by the edge of the bath, still feeling buoyant in my belly from the water. But also having my back accessible to my partner to provide massage for my lower back when I needed it.

When I reflect on my births at home in water, one of the things that is really passionate in my mind is that beautiful smooth transition from being inside you. Being calm, baby swimming up out of the water into your arms. That gaze of seeing your baby for the first time and that wonderful smooth transition from being inside you and then welcoming them into your family. It's amazing, it's calm and it's a beautiful gift that you can give your baby.

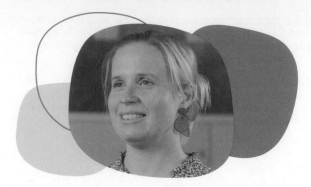

CHAPTER 18

Elise's story

My name is Elise. I'm a midwife and I currently work in a continuity of care model, providing care and births for women in a standalone birth unit as well as home birth.

So, when a woman arrives at the birth centre and you're considering a water birth, the important thing to start with is have the bath at a temperature that is safe for water birth which is between 36.5 and 37.5. And also at a level where the woman is submerged under the water for birthing. So, when you're doing a water birth, a woman can't birth half in/half out. So, you're looking at around nipple line if they're sitting as a basis for where you would like the water. And if they are kneeling, it needs to be the mid back so that their bottom is fully submerged under the water.

When setting up for a water birth, there are certain pieces of equipment that are really important. The main ones that you will need obviously are a thermometer, a doppler, mirror, torch. Women get quite thirsty and dehydrated in labour so it's important to have some water for them. Also, being mindful that they need it to be easy access. So, a straw or a top that's easy for them to drink, because often they're in positions where they can't tilt their head back to get a good drink. They will get really hot, so a fan is really good as well.

Also, when thinking about a water birth, we're in a birth centre. So, the environment is really important. So, when a woman comes in in labour, you don't want their natural role of labour to stall by having bright lights and loud music and all those things happening. So, we have low mood lighting. You might have some aromatherapy going, some candles, if you have access to something that you can pour water over their lower back, whether that's a jug or whether you have a handheld shower that you can use. But because they do get hot, we often use a bowl of ice so that they can have cold flannels on their face or the back of their neck. You will also need a doppler to auscultate the fetal heart. And you need to do that every 15 minutes in first stage for 60 seconds after a contraction. And then in second stage, it's after every contraction or 5 minutes for 60 seconds, whatever comes first basically.

When a woman is labouring in water, particularly the bath, you need to be mindful of their temperature. So, we recommend that you take the woman's temperature every hour when they're in the bath. And be mindful that whatever the woman's temperature is, that the baby's temperature will be a degree higher than that.

When labouring in water, it's important to keep the water clean. So, where possible, we empty the water and top it up with fresh water. It's also important to have something handy that you can scoop foreign objects out of the water if need be. And dispose of those appropriately.

Ideally, you would have your environment ready and your equipment all set up prior to the woman arriving in the birth centre. But if not, you would set up as quickly as possible, and then take a step back and hold that space so that the woman can then labour undisturbed.

From a midwife's perspective, what I really love about water births is that women are really calm in the water. It's a great pain relief option for them. They can get into positions that are more beneficial for them. It's contained, as far as mess goes. It means they can catch their baby in a way where they feel safer, because the baby is more buoyant and they kind of just swim up to the top and they can easily pick them up. They're not worried about dropping them.

And I don't have to wash the baby, it's clean.

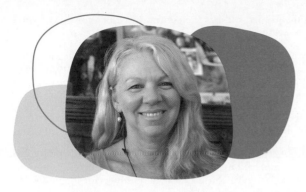

CHAPTER 19

Sheryl's story

My name's Sheryl Sidery. I've been a midwife for 28 years and I'm an independent midwife.

Becoming an independent midwife

So I got into private practice probably only a couple of years after finishing my training. So when I was doing my training at the local hospital, I was always the midwife who was crying up the back of the room. I think a lot of people interpret that, because birth is very beautiful and happy. But really I was crying because I was actually quite horrified at most of the births that I saw.

In the 80s, the caesarean section rate was a lot less than it is now, but it's mainly because Kielland's rotation forceps deliveries was very popular back then. So a lot of women were in stirrups having episiotomies and having their babies turned and pulled out. And I remember just being so shocked and feeling like this just didn't seem like that's how births should be.

And so, right towards the end of my training, I was working with a midwife who I'd never met before. She'd just started working at the hospital and she started speaking to the women in a way that I'd never heard in the, like, 9 months that I'd been there. It wasn't that the other midwives were doing their job badly, but they were just, they were doing things to women, rather than actually just being with them.

And I knew that there was a different way but I didn't know what that way was. And so I started following this midwife around. I'd rearrange my roster so I could work with her. Anyway, we ended up working together for the next 25 years and we became very close friends and wonderful colleagues together.

And it was just a simple thing that she first said, that I remember her saying, 'Just listen to what your body's telling you', and it was the first time I'd heard language like that.

And I was just craving for information on how to be with women in the most effective and beneficial way for the woman. And that seemed to be doing homebirths. So I was very lucky that I was able to get a job at the birth centre at the Royal, so I actually worked there for about 25 years, as well as doing private practice.

But a year ago I decided to leave the public system. It was a quite a brave move but, yeah, I just wanted to see what it would be like to just do this, to just do private practice. And essentially, I'll never look back. It's a way of life, it isn't a job. It doesn't feel like a job at all. It's just it is who I am and I'm absolutely loving it.

We wanted for women to be able to access Medicare to get a rebate for some of their care, but also so that midwives could write their own pathology forms, or to ultrasound and ultimately be able to write prescriptions for the drugs that are necessary to do with birth. So that's only very recently come about.

So for years before, I used to have to get someone else to write all those forms. I used to have a local GP that the women could go to and get all that ordered. So it's not only made it much better for women, but it's opened up an incredible future for midwives to be able to go into private practice. 'Cause, let's face it, that's what the evidence tells us—that if women had their own midwife from the beginning of the pregnancy right through, not only is it public health strategy, 'cause more women end up breastfeeding and have normal births, but there's much more maternal satisfaction and it's a much nicer way for midwives to work.

So because of eligibility now, ultimately what the other thing that will happen is that it will mean that midwives will get visiting rights into the local hospitals.

So that's the next hurdle, is once we get visiting rights it means that women can be offered a range of birth options. Either they can birth-in at home or the birth centre if they have any kind of risk factor, that, where it's safer to birth in hospital they can have their midwife.

So part of being an eligible midwife means having a collaborative arrangement with an obstetrician. And I'm incredibly fortunate and very grateful to have a wonderful relationship with an obstetrician. It's quite a mutual relationship actually; I mean sometimes he will ring me and ask me things about women he might be caring for.

So being able to have that relationship with him means that the woman still has the continuity, which for them is vital and an incredibly satisfying way to work for me, yeah. It's very, very lucky to have that with him.

So, the benefits of midwives now having Medicare eligibility are, financially, it opens it up to more women. The other benefit is that once midwives have access to visiting rights in hospital, it means that there's more likely that midwives could start working in private groups together and be able to just bulk bill women who genuinely can't afford it. And so that gives women so much more choice.

When you look at the research on continuity, the outcomes are far greater. So, I mean I've only got to look at my own statistics to know that just by women choosing this care, they have a far greater chance of having a normal birth. And far less intervention.

So accepting that birth is normal, of course doesn't mean that complications don't ever arise. So it's really important to do, I undertake mandatory training every year for emergency skills. And I think that's really important for midwives. And I think that midwifery practice review that the college offers is also a vital step to ensuring that midwives are reflective on their practice.

So we keep statistics every year and then we collate them and then reflect back on those statistics and MPR provides an opportunity for us to meet with a professional body and provide evidence that our practice is safe.

So, if that's important, which let's face it, we know that it is, having a normal birth has far-reaching consequences for the mother and her infant when we're talking about maternal infant attachment. Then having a normal birth and being able to breastfeed in the first year is really essential. And that's what the evidence tells us.

Working in independent practice

I choose to work in this way because it's just incredibly satisfying. I can have really meaningful relationships with the women because I follow them through from the beginning, right through to when their baby is 2 months old.

A day in the life of an independent midwife

What's the day in the life of a private practising midwife? To be honest, most days you really have no idea. So it's very much about staying in the minute all the time.

Certainly I could wake up in the morning and look at my diary—now I've got three antenatal visits and then a postnatal visit. But if I had a birth overnight, then that would change that, so it's about being really flexible. I mean, it's interesting. Sometimes I could work a couple of hours a day for a few weeks in a row, but then I might have 5 days where I don't have any visits. Actually, that doesn't happen very often.

But look, it doesn't feel, it almost doesn't feel like work, like it feels like, when my phone goes or I'm going to see someone, it's women that I know and I have a relationship with. So it doesn't feel like I'm going to work, like we know each other.

That's the other really wonderful thing about working in this way is that your parameters of normal, well my parameters of normal, expand every year. Because I get to work with families and see things each year that I haven't seen before and realise that it's all normal.

And that we pathologise stuff so much, 'cause if you don't have a relationship with someone how do you know whether what they're feeling or doing is normal or not. But if you know them because you've worked with them for the whole pregnancy and into the postnatal period, you know that, what's normal for them 'cause I know who she is. Like we really know each other. There's an enormous sense of trust.

I know they can give birth without me even being there. And I know that particularly if you look at the evidence, it does say that for low-risk women, homebirth not only is, it's as safe as birthing in hospital, but the maternal satisfaction is far greater. So I really do believe it's the best start for a family, to birth at home. Having said that, sure you can have a wonderful birth in hospital, but I really do think that women have an enormous head start if they have a relationship with someone that they know.

Most satisfying thing about being an independent midwife

Probably the most satisfying thing about working in this way for me is the relationships that I build with the woman and her partner, and then ultimately their children because I've been very fortunate over the years to be their midwife for all of their children.

I mean, ultimately there's such an enormous potential for transformation for women. The whole process of pregnancy is preparing her to become a mother. And for him to become a father, so I mean, I don't facilitate that, but I get to stand by and watch that happening in real time every day.

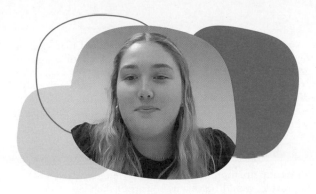

CHAPTER 19

Ella's story

So, my name is Ella. I am a third-year bachelor midwifery student.

Meeting the mother

In my second year of studies I was engaged in a continuity of care experience with a woman who had reached out for student continuity. She was around 12 weeks when we first met. So, it was nice because it was quite early on that we were able to meet. So, she was pregnant with her third baby at the time. And she had found out at an early scan that her baby had a congenital anomaly. It's called anencephaly. So, it's a neural tube defect.

Lots of the time, unfortunately, with anencephaly the babies don't make it and women have miscarriages. However, this baby stayed nice and put and she was able to carry him until 37 weeks. So, throughout her pregnancy we saw lots of different health professionals, lots of different doctors.

There was minimal continuity of care from health professionals at the hospital. She didn't actually have her booking and visit with the midwife until 27 weeks, which is quite late to be having a booking and visit. So, she wasn't engaged into midwifery care as such until around that 27-week mark. Before then it was lots of doctor visits, lots of scans and lots of discussions about whether she was going to keep her baby, or if termination was on the cards at all. And the couple decided to keep their baby. There was a low chance of him surviving once he was born. But they were OK with that chance.

Connecting with baby

So, I would check in with her afterwards. I clearly remember one appointment with the doctor where she messaged me to say that the doctors hadn't even mentioned that her baby had anencephaly. They didn't even have a feel of her baby, or listening to the heart rate, which I think is really important because her baby is still there. It's still her baby. And hearing the heartbeat, regardless of whether or not the baby has a congenital anomaly or not helps you build that connection.

Planning for birth

So, we had a … quite a lengthy discussion about how we would plan for her labour, and birth. We had to have discussions about fetal monitoring, whether or not we would do a CTG, whether or not we would do Doppler's. And if we heard something that wasn't reassuring, would we put a CTG on. Things like that. Also, neonatal resuscitation, whether or not he was going to be fed, yeah. So, we also figured that we would need paediatric input. So, she … I guess my role after that was to go and have a conversation with continuity woman and ask her to write down a list of her wishes and what she would like to happen so that she was part of her … really part of her care. And that we would try to … and support and help her in any way that we could.

Postnatal care

So, when I went to visit her on the postnatal ward the next morning, she had had a normal vaginal birth with her baby. And unfortunately, he passed away after three hours post birth. So, she had—she was rooming in with him in the cuddle cot in the room, and had lots of visitors, and lots of family come up to visit throughout the three days that she stayed on the ward. We did lots of little things to keep the memories alive of him. So, we did hand- and footprints. We did—so we did have a little bit of hair that we could keep that we did pop into a book as well. He had a little bit of hair on the bottom of his—the back of his scalp but given that all the top was open and exposed so there was none at the top. And they had a photographer come and do family photos while they were on the ward. She also had the option to take the cuddle cot home with her and have him at home for as long as she wanted to. However, they just—they chose to just stay in the hospital for the time being and the father also stayed overnight with them as well. So, they did leave after three days. We did link her in as well with social work for further support. And she was going to see her GP for most postnatal support as well. So, on the day that they were leaving I made sure I was there to say goodbye. I guess you've been in their relationship partnership with them for quite a long time, so you've really gotten to know them and it's nice to be there when they leave. So, they—the family didn't want to leave him just in the room on the ward by himself when they left. So, they had asked if they could leave him in my arms when they were leaving, to take care of him. So, that was—that was very much an honour, also a big responsibility to make sure that he was in the best hands possible.

Reflection

So it was definitely a very valuable experience as a student. Not many registered midwives had even had that kind of experience before, especially in a regional town. So, I guess the main things I would take away is that she's still a woman who is pregnant with her baby, and she still requires support and midwifery care throughout her pregnancy, access to continuity of care, which is the gold standard. It shows lots of benefits and would have been great for her not to have to retell her story to every single professional that she saw. The other thing I took away from it was to also take care of yourself as a healthcare professional. It was a lot – it was a lot to take home and I'm very grateful that I had the experience, but you definitely need to have support through that whole time, including antenatally.

On reflection

I think having the plan gave her a little bit of a control back over the situation. And her wishes were respected and we made sure that anything she needed or wanted that we could provide, would be able to be part of the plan.

Final thoughts

So, unfortunately, stillbirth and neonatal loss is part of a midwife's role. And essentially as a midwife we need to ensure that the woman receives the best care possible throughout a very emotional transition and time in her life, not only her life but also her family.

A really nice quote I heard in terms of women carrying babies that have congenital anomalies is that their babies are deemed as incompatible with life, but not incompatible with love. So, they deserve all the love that any other baby would and I'll always be a part of that woman's journey into motherhood and she will remember it for the rest of her life.

CHAPTER 20

Vanessa's story

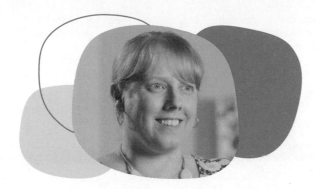

I'm Vanessa and I live in Maitland with my husband and my two daughters who are now 16 and 12 years old, and I had a son called Matthew who would be 13 years old now if he had lived. He was diagnosed with a congenital abnormality called anencephaly when I was 12 weeks pregnant, and we chose to carry him to term.

The diagnosis

In March 2008 I went for a routine ultrasound at 12 weeks. It was my second pregnancy. My daughter was just turned 2 years old at that point and, you know, I had that nervousness of, I haven't really felt that sick this pregnancy, is the baby still alive, what's going to happen? And I went for an ultrasound and the sonographer, you know, showed us the heartbeat and I just thought OK, I'll relax, it's all good. And then towards the end, she said, 'I'm going to have to go and get the doctor.' I thought, 'Oh OK, what's happening here?'

So, she wouldn't actually tell us what was wrong, just that we needed to go and see our GP and we should go straight away. So that was very nerve wracking because we didn't know what was wrong. Just there must be something really badly wrong, but we'd seen the heartbeat, so we were like, what is happening?

So we went to our GP that afternoon and she was the one that told us that our baby had anencephaly and I did know what that word meant. I straight away just thought 'no brain', so yeah, anencephaly is where the brain hasn't fully developed. So, she told us that the baby wouldn't live after he was born and that we had the option to terminate the pregnancy. And my husband was with me, and we sort of looked at each other and said, 'Well, isn't there another option? Can we continue the pregnancy?' And she said, 'Of course, that is the other option, you can continue.'

So that was the diagnosis day. We then went, maybe a week later, to the tertiary hospital to have the diagnosis confirmed. And that was an interesting experience. I guess we'd had a week to look up more about what anencephaly was, read a bit about it. There was a good website at the time that had quite a lot of information for parents, from other parents. And it became clear that not many pregnancies continue to term when the baby has anencephaly. Because they will die either during the pregnancy or shortly after or during the birth or shortly after birth.

So, we went to the tertiary hospital to have another ultrasound. And I remember at that occasion, the obstetrician came to have a look at what was happening, and he wasn't particularly kind about things. He said, 'So what have you been told?' And I said that the baby has anencephaly and he said, 'Well, I'd agree with that' and left the room.

Thankfully, we had a lovely midwife also looking after us that day who gave us options for who else we might want to speak to.

We made it clear that we still intended to carry the baby to term, and so she allowed us to talk to the neonatologists and other people so that we could learn a bit more about what the outcome would be, what services we would need and not need. And we also talked to the obstetrician.

Pregnancy care

Apart from the one poor experience we had with the doctor at the second ultrasound, we generally had a really good experience of care.

So, our GP had written a really great referral letter that made it very clear that our intention was to continue the pregnancy, and I think that was really helpful.

And we … I did shared care, so went and saw the midwives just, I think it was twice during the pregnancy, or saw the obstetrician, I guess more because of this more high-risk situation. I had shared care with my GP who we had known for a long time, and so generally had a really good experience.

One of the things we did at hospital was … we had an actual meeting with their, sort of head midwife and the obstetrician who I was under, and possibly some other members of the team in the birthing suite to discuss our birth plan. And we were able to talk to them about that in detail about what we wanted. You know, we generally wanted as little sort of intervention as possible, and they really respected our wishes.

I heard from somebody years later who was in the room where the … sort of the birth plan was presented to the whole staff and she said that it was just handled so respectfully and kindly. And that was certainly the impression we had of the staff at the hospital, that they were willing to accommodate whatever our wishes were for the birth.

Decision to continue the pregnancy

Reactions to our decision to continue the pregnancy were primarily positive. Yeah, and I think in terms of the reactions that other health professionals had, I really felt that our GP's referral letter, that so eloquently outlined that we had plans to continue the pregnancy … I felt like that really smoothed the way. Because there was no … I was never really challenged on that decision. And I think that was really helpful because we did feel very strongly about it.

We didn't want to negotiate whether we should terminate or not. We were told at the beginning that that was an option. And then we chose to take the other option and that was really respected.

And I think that was very important in making the journey a good one because we, you know, after the initial shock of course of that diagnosis, we then tried really hard during that pregnancy to celebrate our baby's life. So, once we found out he was a boy, we named him Matthew and that name was the name his father had when he was a child. He'd had his name changed as a young child, but Matthew was his father's name originally.

And you know, we try to, you know, do things to remind us of that time when we had Matthew in our lives.

So, our friends and family were very supportive of that decision and helping us to celebrate the life that I had, even if it was just for a short time, yeah.

The birth

Yeah, so when Matthew was born, we knew that because of his anencephaly, it was highly unlikely that I was going to go into spontaneous labour. That seems to be the pattern for these babies. And I knew from some of my own research that the fetal brain is probably involved in the mechanism of labour starting.

So, we had to eventually choose a day for him to be born. And, you know, because of the situation, we were able to choose any time. And we thought, OK, well, our daughter had been born four days late, so we planned for Matthew to also be born four days late. We just thought, OK, we'll do 40 + 4. That's the same as what Annabelle had been born.

So, I was induced. And I think that knowing that the birth plan … we had gone through our plans with the relevant doctors and midwives at the hospital. You know, it was all a very calm process. They were prepared. They often don't get that preparation when a baby is going to die. So, for them, they knew this was coming, but they also had had time to prepare for this situation.

When I went into the hospital that morning, I felt very calm about what was happening. I was ready. We had two fantastic midwives that morning who really looked after us. They gave us, you know, the nicest room, nicest birthing room and got the induction started.

Unfortunately, it didn't seem to do much, so I had the … the drip dose was going up and up and up and nothing was happening. And at some point in the day they examined me, and my waters hadn't actually … my waters hadn't broken and really nothing was happening. So they said, 'Let's break the waters'.

Well, as soon as that happened it was all on because I had been on the highest dose for hours and it was like, right this baby is … this is happening right now.

So, one thing that was interesting was that Matthew was born at just after 3.40 in the afternoon and, so it was around the time of shift change and one of the midwives that had been with us all morning … it was actually her very last day of work, she was retiring. And both the midwives that were on the morning shift stayed to see Matthew be born. And then of course we had the new lot of midwives come in.

So, there were a lot of people in the room.

My husband wanted to deliver Matthew himself and so the midwife who was in charge of that part of the day, she very kindly, you know, talked him through the process and let him be the one to deliver Matthew.

Matthew was born face first, which was a lovely view for everyone to get first rather than his deformity. And the doctor just stood in the background. I knew he was there. But everyone just let it be what we wanted it to be. And there was, you just felt the support of all these people.

And so yeah, my husband delivered Matthew. He was born with a heartbeat but didn't really make any noise. It was very quiet.

I was stunned by how beautiful he was. I think I'd been a bit worried about what he might look like.

But it … and obviously he didn't look like other babies, but to me it was just so beautiful. And, you know, we just got to spend time with him in that moment. Very discreetly someone would come over and check on his heartbeat. And they'd kind of wander off, and you knew they were just keeping tabs on what was happening.

Yeah, and he died in my arms while I was being stitched up. Which is kind of strange, but I didn't know he had died. They told us later, like, oh, we think it was about an hour.

They just let us have time with him. And it wasn't until he was being bathed with my husband and they were dressing him, that Chris said, 'He's gone, hasn't he?' And the midwife said, 'Yeah.'

They were just so lovely about just letting it be our time with him, yeah.

Support offered

I think the biggest thing that helped us through this, you know, undoubtedly the hardest time of my life … the biggest thing that helped us was the support, the respect of the decision we had made to carry to term and the support that we were offered. We were offered every kind of support imaginable.

We saw a perinatal psychologist. And she was kind of like, I'm not sure why you're here, but it was just … and we took on every support we were offered. We saw a social worker at the hospital, and she helped me afterwards with all the paperwork. At that time there was the baby bonus and you had to fill in all these forms for Centrelink and she was there to help with that.

We got to talk to a paediatrician, you know, and there was really nothing he was going to be able to do. But they said, 'Would you like to meet with the paediatrician?' and we said, 'Yes'. Because for all we knew, Matthew could have lived for days, maybe even weeks. And so there was a bit of uncertainty about what sort of care he might need, had he lived longer.

Same with the NICU people. They said, 'You know what, there's nothing we can do, you don't really need the NICU', but they were happy to talk about it and talk it through with us.

So, I think just having … we were offered so much support from all aspects of the system. You know, from the GP to the midwives, the doctors, various people, social work. It was just fantastic to have that level of support around us.

I also chose to seek out support. So, SIDS and Kids as it was called at the time, which now is Red Nose, they were fantastic. I had turned up at their office while I was still pregnant and said, 'My baby is going to die.' They didn't know quite what to say. That was a little unusual, but they were there. You know, I said, 'I'm here to get some resources for my daughter and to think about how to explain this to her.'

It was a very unusual situation.

The funeral directors weren't that great. One of them particularly was not great at understanding, because obviously we had time to prepare for Matthew's death ahead of time, which most women who lose a baby at birth don't have that preparation. And we did, and we chose to use that to really think about what would be next.

And yeah, it was just having people that were willing to just come alongside us and be there and support us in whatever way we thought we needed was really, really, really key.

And, you know, after Matthew died and we had our family come in … my parents brought my 2-year-old in, you know, they brought her ice cream. And she still says like, 'I sat on a purple stool and ate ice cream that the midwife gave me.' Like that was her memory of what happened.

And they allowed us to stay in the room where Matthew was born, for, I think we stayed two nights. Because he was born in the afternoon. You know, they let us stay there. They didn't make me go to the maternity ward. They let us just stay in that room. They brought a bed in for my husband. They made sure we had food because that's not a regular thing in the delivery suite.

And, you know, they let us see Matthew as often as we wanted to. Sometimes he got taken away and then my husband would go and get him and bring him back and things like that. But they let us just take our time.

So, the second day we just spent with him, and some other family came to visit and things like that. And then on the third morning we said 'OK, we're ready to go now', but we were never pushed to leave. Or it was all in our own time and that was really, really good. And you always felt like everybody knew what was happening. No one was caught off guard by our situation because it had been communicated so well throughout that team.

155

The other thing that was really special to us was that a couple of the midwives and the doctor actually came to Matthew's funeral and that was really special. They didn't have to do that. I'm sure it was difficult for them.

And we were aware this is not the kind of day they want to have when they come to work. They don't need these kind of days in their lives and I'm sure they don't want them. But they just stepped into the story with us and walked with us. Even to the extent of coming to the funeral and I'll never forget that.

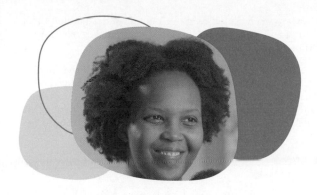

CHAPTER 21

Emma's story

My name is Emma. I'm from Burundi. I have been in Australia for 17 years. I'm married to my husband Idi, and we have two kids. My son is 16 months and my daughter is 3 weeks.

Expectations

My expectation about maternity care in Australia … I would say I didn't honestly know much about it, due to the fact that I don't have any family in Australia who has given birth, for example.

I didn't have any expectation about maternity care in Australia. All I just knew was that the health system here is good, so therefore everything must be good.

Birth experience

My childbearing experiences for my two pregnancies were both different. So, different and the same at the same time I would say, in a way. They were both carried during COVID, so that's the common denominator. Which means that everything was difficult, and appointments were hard. And you couldn't have any support person with you, for example.

But I would say more the first one, because obviously it was the first pregnancy, I had never, sort of, actually been in any health situation in Australia. I had never been to a hospital or anything. So, having to do things through Zoom, for example. Midwifery support through Zoom, that was hard because being the first pregnancy, didn't know what to expect. But obviously someone trying to tell you how to breastfeed through Zoom, for example, that was hard.

I would say second time around was easier, obviously, because things were getting easier COVID-wise. But obviously, being a second-time mother, I sort of knew a bit of what to expect.

Post-partum

I believe the post-partum period is one that's dealt differently from my culture to Australia. In a way that in Australia, and I'm not saying, this is not in a general way, but the post-partum here is more; you've given birth, then OK, if you're good, you're fine physically and mentally I guess, you're OK to continue your journey and do whatever you're doing … cook, clean.

Whereas in my culture, someone who has given birth, you are actually not allowed to leave your home for the next 3 months. So, for the first 3 months of you giving birth, you stay at home. You have your, I guess, you have an army of people around you. Someone cooking, someone cleaning, someone doing this. Literally, all you have to do is just stay in bed and feed.

So, very different, the stage of post-partum. The beginning, the pregnancy, and the rest of it, I would say my culture … there's not much difference between my culture and what I've seen here. It's just that period of post-partum.

The positives

The positives I received during the care, from beginning to end, I would say it's the follow-through of the midwives. Any question that I had, I could ask, and it was OK to ask that question. Because I do believe that in my culture, for example, there are some questions that you are not allowed to ask the medical team. You have to go and ask your mum or aunties.

So, definitely one of the main positives I found with the care here, is the fact that you can easily ask any question to anyone. As in, the medical team. You didn't have to fear anything, yeah.

The challenges

The challenges with being here in Australia as a non-English speaker … there is so much assumptions. So many assumptions are made. And what I realise, now this is something that I've been here for 17–18 years now, it just comes with the fact that you don't speak English and you have a really strange name, therefore you probably don't understand English. Or the English that we're going to be talking about, the 'medical'.

So, the challenges that I experienced was that I think there was so much prejudice about me not understanding them. But I understood them fine. It's more the way they were trying to give out the information if that makes sense. And I guess it's the fact that simply because I'm not from an English-speaking country. Maybe.

The main challenge with both pregnancies was the fact that I couldn't have my husband with me. In any of the appointments. That actually, anyway it's a long story. But the fact that my husband was only, he was stuck overseas for the first pregnancy up until 5 weeks before my son was born. So, which gave me all sorts of anxiety because I was wondering if I was going to give birth by myself. So, in my country, back home for example, I know the husbands don't attend the birth. But they're mostly at the appointments, like the pre-natal appointments. And being here by myself I believed that was a big, yeah, that was a huge challenge.

The support that I've been able to have is nothing compared to what I would have back home. Obviously, it's just by myself here. I don't have any family members, neither does my husband.

Back home you would have, like I've said, an army of people. Your neighbours, your friends, your aunties, your uncles. Like, everyone. Here the support was just from the medical team. And that's usually just the first 5 days and the rest was just my husband. Yeah, so that's it.

Potential improvements

I think it's just the education, like everything. The medical staff educating themselves with the different cultures. And also, don't make assumptions. No make assumptions that 'ohh yes, she's …'. Because I know there was a comment that was made in the ward. I remember now. It was like 'oh African women, oh you are known for being so strong, you will get through this'. This is after 15 hours of labour. 'You will be fine with this, you are African are known for this'. Africa is not a country so there's about 50 something countries there. We're not the same. We're not meant to be the same. Everyone is different. It's a different culture, like everyone has their different cultures. So, educate yourself.

I believe the main what can be done, the main thing is to educate the medical team. And yeah, just learn. No make assumption.

CHAPTER 21

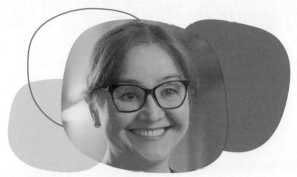

Sabera's story

My name is Sabera and I'm from Afghanistan originally. I'm a midwife and I studied my midwifery in Iran during war when we migrated to Iran. I completed my education in Iran. And later on, I came as a refugee to Australia, and I studied my PhD here in Australia. Recently I'm working as a research fellow with the University of Technology Sydney.

My research topic is female genital mutilation, and how we can provide quality of care to women who have undergone female genital mutilation, or so-called FGM, the abbreviation.

I came across this topic when I came in Australia. And I started my work with the university as a researcher. There was a project which was looking at the health system, how they deal with these women who have undergone female genital mutilation and migrated to Australia. And also, we look at the prevalence of FGM in area which is concentrated with population who migrated from those countries which this practice is highly prevalent.

But at the time, what inspired me to this research was that the whole scenario was one-sided. The whole project was focused on the health system and the views of providers, without looking at the other side of the story, which was women who were receiving this care. And I decided to do my study on experience and needs of women who have undergone female genital mutilation and migrated to Australia; what is their experience, what they regard as quality of care? Yes, we define quality of care from health system views. But is that really what woman wanted? And I bring these two concepts together to see how much that our definition matching the woman's desire and wishes. That's my research.

According to the World Health Organization, female genital mutilation, or so-called as abbreviation FGM, is total or partial removal of external female genitalia for non-medical purposes. According to WHO, there are different types of FGM from Type-1 to Type-4. Which is, that Type-1 is the mildest and as we go further it's severe. The Type-2 is the most common type, and the Type-3 is called infibulation, which they literally cut everything; clitoris, labia. And at the end stitch the external female genitalia all the way down and just remain a hole for urination and menstruation.

What we find in this research is mostly based on the experience and women's views on quality of care. And what they desire. What we found, that the communication is so poor when these women goes through the maternity services in Australia. And there are lots of cultural and language barriers in receiving quality of care in maternity services within Australian health system.

These women also think that they didn't receive the level of … they appreciate the care they received in Australia because they feel they are safer. And all the emergency facilities are available to them if there is something going wrong. But at the same time also, they acknowledge that the level of quality was not what they expected or they desired. Most of the time they faced the cultural and communication barriers. For example, their language was not understood by the health providers and their culture, cultural understanding was really, really important to them.

Most of these women I saw think that they were isolated from decision making during their care. And they were not part of the decision making. Maybe the communication was the reason, but some of them mentioned that they found themself in a middle of operation room without knowing what they were going to do on them. For example, the health provider decided that this woman should be deinfibulated. But they took the woman to the operation room without properly or clearly communicating with woman what we are doing for you or why you are here. That was a big challenge for woman. And most women which, in my study, they talk about those kind of things; that they were not properly involved in decision making and design of their care. That's what they want. They want to be co-designer of their care.

Get as much as information and self-learning about this topic as you can. And make your understanding of the culture clear. This culture might be very brutal and negative in your eye as a health professional, but it's highly respected for woman as a part of their culture or religion. You shouldn't regard it as a disrespectful practice when you communicate with woman.

Then, communication is key. You need to be very, a very professional communicator when you deal with these groups of women. Because the subject is very sensitive and the words even you use … for example, in some culture if you use words 'cutting' instead of female genital mutilation, it's very disrespectful.

Training or being educated yourself, it doesn't mean to go to a classroom and see. There are plenty of resources and material available through UN agencies and we also developed an e-learning module for health professionals to guide them during their practice. Plenty of material out there to guide you how to react and how to deal with those women during maternity services. Plus, each midwife definitely should know about legal aspects of FGM practice in Australia. Because that might determine the next pathway for a woman on what to do with woman when they disclose to you.

And then, protocol and guidelines available within your practice, within the hospitals or clinic you're working. You need to be aware of those things because without knowing those clinical guidelines you might be lost, you might be confused and also you make the woman confused. Because in my research we found that women lost within health system. Because they don't know what is next for them.

No woman will disclose to you in one session what they have been undergone or what happened in their life. You have to have that continuum of care with the woman, especially these groups of women who are very vulnerable, culturally and socio-economically, and in terms of gender-based violence. You need to do that relationship through continuum of care. Not just these women, in all groups of women we need that continuum. Evidence proved that we need continuum of care. For these groups, I definitely advise you to have continuum of care to build a trusting relationship with the woman. And during this relationship you have to empower those women to raise their voice. And also, they look at you as an advocate to support them. Not just in terms of being with them during birth and deliver their baby, but also to support them. Because when we talk about deinfibulation, opening a woman after they've been closed during FGM, which we call it infibulation. This deinfibulation concept is not a small or minor deal for women.

When we talk about dealing with FGM it's not a clinical concept, it's a social-cultural concept. And you need to deal with that aspect, beside the clinical aspect. Yes, you need to learn how to deinfibulate the woman, you need to learn about different types of FGM.

But at the same time, you need to learn how to transfer those knowledge when you deal with the actual community. Like, going to the woman's house, you can get that opportunity to connect with the family and community. Because many of these women are under pressure to do this practice in their young generation like their daughters. You are the key person to prevent that practice in some stage. And not allowing this practice to continue for the next generations. Just by advocating, and talking to people, and get connecting and understanding the culture. And empowering women.

CHAPTER 22

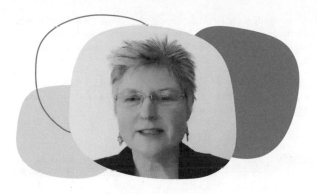

Namira's story

I work currently as CEO in Disability Maternity Care within New South Wales. I've been a midwife for about 30 years, and worked in a variety of midwifery roles. In 2012, I began researching my PhD. And I looked particularly at and studied maternity care for women with an intellectual disability. And that's come from my own lived experience. I have two women in my family who have cognitive impairments, one with an acquired brain injury, and the other has an intellectual disability. They were pregnant and became mums within the early years of my PhD. They had quite different outcomes, one kept a baby and one didn't keep her baby.

Visible and invisible disabilities

So, disability can either be physical disability, it can be from birth such as spina bifida, or it can be an acquired disability such as somebody who has a spinal cord injury. It can also be a sensory disability, so hearing impairment, or a vision impairment, a cognitive impairment, which can either be acquired or from birth, such as intellectual disability. And it can also include mental illness, particularly if it's a lifelong mental illness. The important thing to think about when we think about disabilities is that there are visible disabilities, and there's also invisible disabilities. So, when we think about visible disabilities we're thinking about somebody who is obviously … has a visual impairment, so they may have a guide dog assisting them which becomes apparent to everybody that it's a guide dog, or they may be using a cane, or it might be somebody who is in a wheelchair. So, that's very visible and apparent to everybody. But when we think about invisible disabilities, there are disabilities that really aren't apparent unless we actually start communicating with a person or that they decide to disclose them. So, those sorts of things can be intellectual disability because not everybody looks like they have a disability if they have an intellectual disability. We know that people with Down syndrome have particular characteristics that are visible to the community, but other people with an intellectual disability you may not know until you actually start talking to them. Other invisible disabilities also include things like chronic pain. If somebody has, you know, rheumatoid arthritis that you might not know about it until they actually disclose it to you. So, that's important to think about. And I think the really important thing to think about is, you know, we often talk about a significant disability. So, we need to be thinking about how does a person view their disability. Do they see it as significant? We might think it's significant, but they actually don't see it as very significant. It's only a small aspect of their lives. And again, a person might have what we would consider as an insignificant disability. So, for example, it only might be a mild intellectual disability. So, we think, oh well, that's not too bad. They can talk and do all the rest of it. But it actually contributes to how they actually process information, how they communicate, how they understand information, and it can actually perhaps be a really, really big barrier in their life, particularly if it's combined with other sorts of comorbidities, or perhaps if they've got autism as well, or other mental illnesses, or even, you know, things like anxiety and depression can exacerbate what might be considered as sort of a less significant disability. So, it's really important when we think about disability, we're thinking about it from the person's perspective and we allow them to decide how significant they think it is and how it impacts their life.

Models of care and services

In terms of barriers, there aren't suitable models of care that meet their needs. We don't have specific programs set up generally, there actually is a special Women in Need's clinic in one of the hospitals in Victoria, in Melbourne. But generally, we don't have specific programs for women with disabilities. Often they can be actively excluded from continuity of care programs because they're seen as—too time intensive. Often they have lots of other complex issues in their lives that contribute to their complexity.

Attitudes

A study in 2012 showed that—a third of midwives didn't believe that women with intellectual disability should have children. So, if you have a third of midwives having attitudes like that, then how are they actually going to support and help those mums learn what they need to learn in order to transition and become a mother? So, addressing some of those attitudes and the stigma that is related to disability is really, really important.

I think most important thing first and foremost is listen to the woman. Listen to what she's telling you, what her needs are. You know? I know we talk about women-centred care in midwifery. It is really important we provide that when we're working with a woman who has a disability. So, listening to how she sees herself, how does she see her disability impacting on her life and potentially impacting on her mothering abilities?

There's some amazing mums out there who have limb deficiencies, and they do amazing jobs of actually, looking after their babies, changing their babies. They know what they can do and what they need help with. So, it's really important that we listen to them, we see them as the experts of their own health and their own abilities.

Flexibility

The other important things are having flexible practices within hospitals. So, rather than say, 'Yeah, no, our policy is that partners, you know, particularly if they're men they can't stay overnight. It's just our policy that they don't do it. We can't make an exception. For many women with disabilities, you know, statistically we know that at least half of them probably have anxiety and depression. So, taking them away from their main supports and having them in hospital for however many days it might be, they're actually going to have an incredible amount of anxiety around that. And if you think about that in terms of a woman who has an intellectual disability who is struggling already to understand information that's presented when a person has anxiety it actually decreases their ability to understand information, whether they have an intellectual disability or not. So, why not allow their main support people to be with them 24 hours to actually provide that emotional support for them, but also to provide the physical support they might need? They're going to be the people who are actually supporting that mum at home and helping her develop her skills. So, they need to be learning how that mum has actually been given the information in hospital, so they can continue providing the information and support in the same way.

The birthing mother

I think that's really important is that we recognise the birthing mother. No matter what circumstances are, we know that two out of three women with an intellectual disability, will probably have their babies removed either following birth, or at some point when there's a crisis sort of down the track probably in that, you know, first couple of years of life, and they lose care of their baby. We know from the Stolen Generation and from research around adoptive children how important that birthing mother is, how important that connection is for those adults when they become adults. So, we need to recognise that. And we need to enable every opportunity for that mother to have a connection at some point, you know, whether she—you know, even if she can't look after her baby full time, how can we enable her to be part of that baby's life on a regular basis so that that baby as they grow into adulthood, they do have regular contact with their birthing mother? And we need to honour that role that those birthing mothers have. The other things I think that are important that we need to consider are that, you know, and I was talking a bit about it before, where we have flexible hospital practices, but we also need to remember that … how important is … everybody learns differently. If a mum has a learning or an intellectual or learning disability, it's going to take her longer to learn those mothering skills. And we need to be able to give her the time to be able to do that. And I think the take-home message is that we need to be walking beside them. We need to be enabling them through recognising their own expertise, through recognising that they can make decisions in their lives rather than trying to take over and make decisions for them.

Interdisciplinary care

In terms of a story, I'd like to tell you the story about Suzie. I was working in the antenatal clinic at the time. And Suzie was about 40 years old and she had a mild intellectual disability and she also had cerebral palsy. She walked with a— portable walker. She previously had had two children about ten and eight years previously, and both those children had been removed from her care and were in foster care. Suzie had been seeing one of the obstetricians. And the obstetrician thought that the clinic would be much better to facilitate Suzie's care. So, I became involved in Suzie's care. I must say, Suzie had a fantastic sense of humour and it was always really enjoyable spending time with Suzie. Suzie was really keen to keep this baby because of the trauma that had happened with her other two children. We were able to actually provide some degree of continuity. Most of her antenatal care, I had seen her. We made accommodations to her—rather than being necessary, just staying at the clinic, which unfortunately at that time didn't have a height-adjustable bed, she actually had to come up to the birthing unit to have her antenatal checks. Which she was happy to do, but again that's another thing that needs to be addressed, you know, looking at actually how we provide equipment to women within the hospital doesn't actually meet their needs. Suzie, you know, we had lots of discussion around birthing. And Suzie ended up—I wasn't there for the birth, but Suzie had a normal vaginal birth and she stayed in hospital longer than would be anticipated for a mainstream mum. But she did really well. We had the social worker involved. We had an OT involved. So, we were all looking at different ways that we could actually set her up so when she went home, she had her house and home set up to accommodate her particular needs. And it was great. I actually bumped into Suzie 12 months later and she still had the care of her baby and she was doing really well and her walker had actually been changed so that she could actually have her baby on the walker. So, instead of trying to walk with the walker, as well as having the baby, her walker had sort of been changed so that she could have the baby carried on the walker. Yeah. And she was doing really well and really enjoying being a mum this time. So, I think, you know, that shows you how important it is actually looking at what those mums' needs are, accommodating those needs, having continuity of care, having someone who is the main care provider who can actually then link her in with lots of other providers that she would need to meet her needs.